Scripts and Strategies in Hypnotherapy Volume II

Roger P. Allen Dp Hyp PsyV

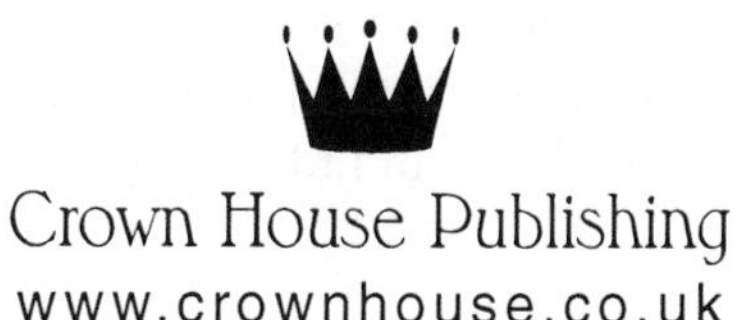

Crown House Publishing
www.crownhouse.co.uk

First published in the UK by

Crown House Publishings Limited
Crown Buildings
Bancyfelin
Carmarthen
Wales
SA33 5ND
UK

www.crownhouse.co.uk

British Library of Cataloguing-in-Publication Data
A catalogue entry for this book is available from the British Library.

ISBN 1899836691

Typeset by Mac Style Ltd, Scarborough, N. Yorkshire
Printed and bound in the UK by
Bell & Bain Ltd, Glasgow

Dedication

This book is dedicated to the memory
of my father, Leonard Allen.
He survived the horrors of war in Burma
to fall at the age of 56 years to the effects
of tobacco addiction.

Table of Contents

Foreword

After the huge success of *Scripts and Strategies in Hypnotherapy*, so many people asked me whether I intended to follow that book with another. Initially, I was not enamoured with the idea. After all, putting together a book that is going to prove useful to therapists who may already have years of experience under their belt is a daunting task.

I came to the conclusion that to produce a work that will continue to serve in the same way as my previous effort, in that therapists will be able to use the content to help with the formulation of therapy sessions, I needed to include the efforts of others in order to ensure that the book covers a broad tranche of ideas and experience.

As before, I am certain that many of the ideas which are included within these pages will prove to be the property of others who have contributed to the vast store of knowledge available within the profession. Wherever possible I have ensured that proper accreditation is given and apologise now for the fact that this really is an impossible task. To those who have contributed and remain anonymous, I extend my thanks and appreciation.

Much of the content has been derived from experience gained during therapy sessions. In order that the ideas put forward are expressed in the best possible way, the therapy session so described is not necessarily one that actually took place but is rather an amalgamation of therapy experiences. It is recognised that no two sessions are ever the same, just as we accept that no two people are the same, as each person experiences in his or her own unique way.

The final session in this book comprises a stop smoking therapy. This is an area in which I have, for the past five years, gained a reputation which brings me many referrals.

My method, evolved over the years, involves a one session therapeutic approach and an appointment with each client that lasts for up to two hours. The whole of the thinking, client conditioning and content, including scripted material, is included in what could be considered a complete course on 'Smoking Cessation'.

I have not involved myself much in the way of psychology and delving into the deeper meaning of the effectiveness of the contents of the following pages. Such material I have kept to a minimum on the huge assumption that you, the reader, are already a practising therapist, having received formal training and possessing qualifications that have given you a good and working grounding in the basic concepts within which we therapists work. I have, however, not been able to refrain completely from expressing just a few of my own ideas.

There are many schools of thought that make up the consensus which accepts hypnosis as a valuable adjunct to therapy, and I am sure that you will find just a little of everything within these pages forming part of the therapeutic approach to each situation.

Should you agree with everything that is written here, then welcome to my world! I recognise, however, that disagreement with the status quo provides the climate for new thinking. This adds to the continuing development of exciting new strategies.

In writing *Scripts and Strategies in Hypnotherapy*, I was very careful to ensure that my readers recognised that the ideas contained within the scripts were to be considered as 'adaptable'.

Much of what happens within the actuality of a therapy session is a response to what is happening with our client, and our own best response is the one that springs from the wealth of knowledge and experience that is accumulated and contained within our own subconscious.

The scripts and the described approaches are all products sourced from within the subconscious as we, as therapists, make appropriate responses to the unique situation that is presented by clients who present unending challenges in that they are all different.

The accumulation of ideas provides us with a vast ready store of data and direction that we can select from and combine in order that each response is appropriate and best suited towards the well being of the client and his or her needs.

Scripted material that is utilised to deal with similar situations in a general and perhaps safe way will often produce good results. Material which is used and adapted to suit a given situation and the uniqueness of a client will go so much further to achieving that rapport with clients which is essential.

The mere mention of some small thing that is significant and important to a client within the language used by the therapist is perhaps that which opens that vital door and makes the therapy effective, e.g. *"I wonder if you can remember just how good you felt when you first held that puppy when you were just ten years old and how special that time was"*.

I have contented myself with a few comments within the text that I consider relevant, that perhaps support the importance of a particular approach. Hopefully I have refrained from allowing my imagination to send me off on flights of fancy, imposing too many of my own sometimes radical opinions upon you, my reader!

Finally, I have referred to my clients in the masculine. This is not in any way intended as sexist but as a means of simplifying the text.

Inducing the Trance State

Inducing hypnosis is not something that can be described as what we "do" to a client. It has been broadly recognised that we as therapists are only instrumental in helping our subject to utilise an ability that everyone possesses, i.e. to go into a trance. Thus, the trance state can be achieved only with the co-operation of the client.

Most people who appear in a therapist's office for the first time already have an impression of what to expect; usually a very flawed expectation that has been generated by seeing a stage hypnotism show, reading a book or seeing a film that depicts hypnosis as some kind of magical influence that can be used to bend mere mortals to our will.

Many people report that becoming hypnotised feels at first like falling asleep, but with the difference that somehow they keep hearing my voice as a sort of background to whatever experience they may have. In some ways hypnosis is like sleepwalking: however, hypnosis is also an individual experience and is not just alike for everyone. In a sense the hypnotised person is like a sleepwalker, for he can carry out various and complex activities while remaining hypnotised. (Weitzenhoffer & Hilgard, 1959)

The concern of many is that they will be subject to anything the therapist wishes to inflict upon them, without their consent. This concern is, of course, unfounded, and the situation needs to be clarified in order to put the client's mind at ease. Most of us have a bank manager, but none of us have been able to persuade him to allow us free use of his golden shovel!

I always explain to my client exactly what hypnosis is in real terms: while watching television, the experience that can result when becoming so engrossed in a particularly good show, where all else in the room just fades into insignificance; when someone can speak to us and not be heard because all our attention is taken up by what is happening on that small screen. Hypnosis is the focusing of the conscious attention within such a narrow corridor of influence. This is the trance state that we are seeking to induce.

When the conscious mind is so intensely focused in this way, the other influences that are present, such as the person who asks if you would like a drink, are no longer being rationalised or critically analysed. The words are heard, but by the subconscious mind free of the critically analytical interference of the conscious mind which, through a process of derivational search, filters out those things which are not acceptable and formulates a perception of events which can then be allowed into the subconscious, in a suitably altered manner. The conscious mind tells us that black is black and, if it receives a suggestion that it is white, then it will intervene to ensure that the correct perception is formed. Without the influence of the conscious mind the subconscious will accept that black is white without objection.

It is for this reason that hypnosis is so useful an adjunct to therapy, as it allows the subconscious resources of the client to be accessed and influenced through suggestion delivered in many forms. Direct or indirect suggestion, imagery etc, the many and various strategies used in hypnotherapy, are simply differing techniques utilised to deliver beneficial suggestions, to change maladaptive learned responses into responses which are adaptive and thereby offer positive options for the client.

Of the many useful works available for those wishing to make a study of trance phenomena, I would suggest that *Hypnosis in Therapy* is a useful addition to the library of any therapist. *(Gibson & Heap ISBN 0-86377-155-6 published by Laurence Erlbaum Associates 1991).* Also *Trancework (Michael Yapko 1990)*

The following inductions are just a few of so many. They are not magical spells, simply forms of words that will assist the client to tap into his own ability to relax and go into trance.

Eyes Sealed Shut
Rapid Induction

It is best if the client is seated in a comfortable chair; I ask him to remove his glasses and loosen any tight clothing so that he can relax in complete comfort.

Okay, now we will do some hypnosis, and I know that you will be wondering whether you will easily go into a trance ... I can tell you now that what will happen is natural and normal as I ask you to utilise your own ability to relax and drift into a very deep state of relaxation ... the state known as hypnosis. It is so very true that provided you just follow the simple instructions that I give to you ... you will drift into hypnosis. Of course ... you can resist me ... but that is not what you came here for ... is it? *(Await response)*

So make yourself very comfortable now ... and just look at a spot on my hand right here as you listen to my voice ... concentrating fully on that spot on my hand ... without allowing your eyes to move away from that spot on my hand ... Very soon, perhaps now ... you will become aware of how heavy your eyes become so quickly ... they will want to blink and that's fine ... perhaps they become a little watery ... or a little dry ... and that's fine too ... they can feel so heavy and so tired ... droopy and drowsy ... and it would be so nice to just allow them to close ... as I bring my hand down slowly ... past your eyes ... past your nose ... past your mouth ... closing ... closing ... and closed now. That's good ... already you are beginning to relax and feel so very comfortable.

Now I am going to touch your forehead with my finger ... here. I am locking your eyes from the outside as you lock them from the inside ... and as I count from one to five you will find them locking tighter and tighter.

One: Eyes tightly closed **Two**: Locking tight and sealing shut. **Three**: Sealing shut as though they were glued. **Four**: The more that you try to open them the tighter they become. **Five**: Now satisfy yourself ... make a try and find them locking tighter and tighter.

Now allow that feeling ... a wave of relaxation ... to flow down through your body ... arms ... legs ... your whole body becoming loose and free as all tension flows from you and you relax deeper ... ever deeper ... with every word that I speak.

Continue with deepener and session.

Age Progression

A technique famously employed by the master Milton Erickson MD He would encourage clients to experience events and situations in the future and then ask them to describe what methods they had employed to deal with the particular problem that was the subject of the therapy.

This would have the effect of allowing the client to experience at a subconscious level having successfully completed making changes that were life enhancing.

'And time can have passed since this time spent here now ... a few days perhaps and then time can pass so quickly ... and then a few weeks ... even months ... since that time you and I spent then ... when you discovered something that was so special to you and how good you felt ... and the way that your thoughts at that time then ... that allowed you to look back at that time before so differently ... I wonder if you can tell me now just what is different from then ... And what can you do that is so much more beneficial that you couldn't do back at that time then ...'

Amnesia

It can be useful for the client not to retain memory of session content if rationalisation could prove detrimental to what has been achieved subconsciously.

As you drift and dream ... continuing to relax in that special way ... breathing easily ... quietly ... relaxing deeper and deeper with every gentle breath ... I wonder if you can recall how much you have concerned yourself with those thoughts ... those fleeting memories of events ... ideas that drift in and out ... The subconscious mind can work so hard when it relaxes too ... and then you can become so aware of how difficult it can be to recall what I was telling you five minutes ago ... And then what if you could remember what I said seven and a half minutes ago ... what you were thinking ... just a minute ago ... or even four minutes ago ... It really can seem to be just too much effort to make ... to try to remember ... not worth the bother ... so much easier to just allow that relaxation ... that comfortable time to continue ... with a knowing that you really have no need at all to concern yourself at all ...

Snippet:-

When asked a question by the therapist, the client replies, "I don't know".

Therapist, "If you did know, what would the answer be?"

Advice is something that a therapist should avoid giving at all costs. To give advice that is compatible with the situation of the client we would first need to be in the client's situation, experiencing exactly as he experiences which is, of course, impossible:

Advice is invariably prefixed by the one phrase that devalues the whole exercise, "If I were you".

We all see the world from our own particular point of view, and, no matter how good we may feel we are at relating to another person's point of view, it will remain that other person's point of view, and not our own.

"I wonder if you are aware, Mary, that good co-operative hypnotic subjects are so easy to spot as they close their eyes just as you are doing now?"

"It can be such a relaxing experience to just allow your eyes to close naturally, wouldn't you agree?"

"Many of my clients tell me that my voice can sound so much more relaxing when you close your eyes. Can you close your eyes now?"

"When you are ready to begin, just allow your eyes to close."

Ticking Clock Induction

If there is a clock in the room this can be utilized with this induction as you suggest that the client concentrate on the ticking of that clock. This, however, is not a necessity, as it can be suggested to the client that a clock be imagined and that the ticking of that clock can be something that suggests relaxation.

Now that you're resting comfortably there ... with your eyes closed ... feeling safe and secure ... I want you to take three very deep breaths and then breathe normally ... So go ahead now ... breathe in ... very deeply ... and now exhale ... Now take a second breath ... inhale ... and exhale. And now ... another ... inhale ... exhale ... Now be aware of your eyes ... how comfortable they feel ... closed ... and just breathe normally.

I want you to concentrate on only my voice now ... putting aside any other thoughts that come to mind ... and I'm going to draw your attention to various parts of your body ... and as I draw your attention to that part ... then I want you to relax every muscle and nerve ... in that part of your body ... as I refer to it in turn.

First of all I want to draw your attention to your fingers ... and your hands ... your wrists ... your forearms ... and your upper arms ... and as you consider this area of your body ... I want you to be aware of any tension in those muscles ... and concentrate on that tension.

Now ... relax all those muscles ... every nerve ... every fibre ... in your hands and arms ... allow all of that tension to flow away ... to drain down ... let those muscle come to rest ... lengthen and loosen ... let them just feel very comfortable ... heavy ... very relaxed ... very ... very relaxed.

And when you have relaxed those muscles in this way ... then I want you to concentrate on your feet ... your ankles ... your calves ... your knees and your thighs ... be aware of any tension in those muscles ... and as you concentrate on them ... then again ... relax every muscle ... every fibre in your legs and feet ... allowing all of that tension to flow away ... to drift down ... lengthening ... loosening ... so that these muscles too feel very loose and comfortable ... heavy ... very ... very relaxed.

Now be aware of your trunk ... your stomach muscles ... and your chest muscles ... and notice too how all the muscles in this part of your body are now becoming more and more relaxed ... lengthening ... loosening ... much more relaxed ... coming to rest as all of the tension just drains away ... draining away now just like the grains of fine sand in an hour glass drain down into the bottom of the glass.

Now be aware of your shoulders ... the muscles in your neck and your scalp ... be aware of the tension here ... and now you can release that tension as every muscle in this part of your body now becomes more and more relaxed ... loosening and lengthening ... very ... very relaxed ... so that you can feel all the muscles throughout your entire body now ... loose ... limp and relaxed ... as that comfortable heaviness continues now.

And while you're resting in this way ... I want you to imagine that it's a beautiful summer's day ... I want you to imagine that you are floating on a cloud ... It's so quiet and peaceful .. and there you are ... at ease with the world ... just drifting and dreaming as you float on and on and ... on and on ...

Now you're feeling very comfortable ... so much at ease and completely relaxed ... and it's such a pleasant feeling ... such a soothing feeling ... a feeling as though you just want to drift far away ... into a deep ... sound ... heavenly sleep ... You're so much at ease ... and every muscle and nerve in your entire body is completely relaxed and at ease ... and you feel so pleasantly heavy ... so completely relaxed ... that you just want to continue in this way ... going into a deeper ... deeper relaxation.

Every part of your body feels so heavy and comfortable ... so easy ... I wonder now if you can just let yourself sink and drift ... deeper ... further into relaxation.

And now I'm going to count from one to three ... and on the count of three ... I want you to have drifted into a much ... much deeper relaxation than the one you are in at the moment.

One. And your entire body is completely relaxed ... every muscle and nerve is completely relaxed and at ease ... and your body feels so heavy. **Two**. Your head feels so heavy and sleepy ... It's a very pleasant feeling ... You feel so heavy and tired ... and you keep falling further and deeper into relaxation ... and your thoughts are vanishing ... All you can do is think of relaxation ... deep ... sound relaxation. **Three**. You are now in a deep ... sound relaxation ... and you'll continue to drift deeper and further ... so that every word I utter will put you into a deeper and sounder sleep ... and all you can hear is my voice. ... You can hear no other sounds ... All the other sounds that surround us ... background noises ... traffic noises ... all of these are insignificant ... you become oblivious to all of these ... because all that is important is the sound of my voice.

Now *(client's name)* ... I want you to become aware of the sound of the clock here in the room ... You can be aware of the steady and relaxing consistency of the ticking of the clock as it marks time.

This ticking of the clock that you are so aware of now ... is going to relax the rhythm of your brain .... and as the rhythm of your brain slows down comfortably ... so then you will drift into a deeper ... and deeper relaxation.

Now I'm going to count from one to seven ... and I shall use the words ... "drift deeper" ... in between each count ... and you'll find that by the time I reach the count of seven ... you will be very deeply relaxed ... very ... very deeply relaxed.

One ... drift deeper ... **two** ... drift deeper ... **three** ... deeper and deeper ... drift deeper ... **four** ... drift deeper ... **five** ... much much deeper into hypnosis ... drift deeper ... **six** ... drift deeper ... **seven** ... and now into a deep ... satisfying and comfortable trance state.

And now I want you to notice that in a few moments ... that you will no longer be aware of that ticking sound ... and when this noise stops ... that the rhythm of your brain will have slowed down to the extent that you will be aware of nothing ... nothing but a beautiful silence ... a complete silence ... a peaceful silence ... in which nothing but the sound of my voice breaks through.

When this noise stops ... you'll be aware of only the sound of my voice ... no other sound will be of any consequence to you ... I want you now to enjoy that silence ... because with this silence ... you have achieved a peace that is yours ... relaxation is yours ... and you can feel yourself in harmony with nature. You can now enjoy peace ... tranquillity and a oneness with your own wise inner mind where all can be resolved and made good.

Continue with therapy session.

Children up to Age 10

Begin in a conversational manner. It can be helpful to find out what is the child's favourite toy.

Now … *(client's name)* ... I expect that you play a lot with your toys at home ... I bet that you have a lot of toys and that when you play with them you pretend that they are real ... don't you? ... I know that I did ... when I was a little boy like you. Well ... you know we have a game of pretend here too ... and if you learn this game with me ... nothing that will happen here today will bother you at all. Would you like to learn this game? ... I know you will. Okay now *(client's name)* ... let's start by taking a big deep breath in ... and then let it all out ... Now you can open your eyes just as wide as you can and I am going to show you this game of pretend. Now I am going to pull your eyelids closed ... like this ... *(finger & thumb technique)* and you can pretend that you just can't open your eyes ... That's all you have to do ... Just pretend as hard as you can that you just can't open your eyes no matter what ... pretend so hard that when you try to open your eyes ... they just won't work at all ... Now try to make them work when you are pretending like that ... the more you try the more they will not work because you are pretending so hard ... and because you are so good at pretending. Nothing that happens now will bother you or disturb you at all ... in your mind ... You can be at home playing with your favourite toys ... and you need not concern yourself with anything else at all ...

Concept: David Elman

Inside/Outside Induction

Ensure that the subject is seated comfortably with eyes closed.

Okay *(client's name)* ... I want you now to begin to breathe in and out in time with me. ... Now take a deep breath in ... Hold it ... Now exhale slowly. *(Repeat 6 times)*

Now relax every muscle and every fibre of your body as completely as you can ... and say inwardly to yourself ...

"I am becoming very relaxed." .... "My eyelids are so relaxed now ... that I cannot open them. I try but cannot open my eyes ... so I am drifting into hypnosis."

(Watch for reaction as client tries to open eyes but finds no response)

"I am drifting down into deep hypnosis. I am becoming so sleepy ... so sleepy ... I am drifting down into deep hypnosis where my subconscious mind will accept every suggestion and put it into action with perfection."

"I am so relaxed that my head is dropping forward onto my chest and I sink into deep hypnosis."

(Watch for response) (Now move emphasis from self hypnosis to your instruction)

"Good ... That's very good ... you are going deeper and deeper into profound hypnosis now. All you have to do is relax and drift down deeper into hypnosis."

Attributed to Dwight Bale.

Arm Levitation Induction

The client should be sitting ... eyes closed ... in a straight chair.

The first thing that I would like you to do ... before you continue to relax ... and enter into a trance ... is to place the very tips of your fingers very lightly ... just touching your thighs ... with your arms in the air and unsupported ... your elbows away from your sides ... just floating there ... fingers barely touching the cloth ... so that you can just feel the texture ... that's right fingers barely touching ... and now focus your attention on those sensations in the very tips of your fingers ... where they barely touch ... where that floating continues ... because as I talk to you ... and you continue to relax ... and to pay close attention to those sensations ... an interesting thing is beginning to happen. Because everyone knows how easy it is to learn something when you are comfortable. And sooner or later everyone has the experience of learning something new when they are relaxed ... so go ahead now and allow that comfortable feeling to continue ... with the recognition that after a while you can notice that your unconscious mind has begun to gently lift up one hand or the other ... or perhaps both. It may be difficult to hold it there ... just barely touching your thigh ... as it keeps trying to move upwards a bit as it feels lighter ... and lighter ... and lifts upwards ... almost by itself at times while the other may seem to get heavier ... difficult to tell the difference at first ... but as you pay close attention ... it becomes easier and easier to notice which seems heavier ... and which seems lighter ... And when you begin to notice which hand seems heavier ... you may let it relax and come to rest comfortably on your thigh ... while you pay more and more attention to that other hand ... to that light upwards lifting hand that moves up a bit at times ... and back down again perhaps ... and then back upwards again. And after a while you may begin to notice that you can allow that drifting upwards to continue ... more and more upwards ... lighter ... floating upwards as you allow that movement to continue on and on ... an automatic movement upwards as your unconscious mind lifts that hand ... that arm ... upwards one step at time ... upwards and then more and more. It may be difficult to tell exactly how much that arm and hand have drifted up ... to tell exactly what position they are in ... and it may be difficult to tell when that slow effortless movement occurs more and more rapidly ... as it drifts up ... lighter and lighter ... higher and higher. That's right *(Pause for upward movement)* ... that's right.

And that hand and that arm can continue to drift higher and become lighter and lighter ... but as you pay close attention to them ... you may begin to notice how they feel now ... how tired and heavy they are ... as your unconscious mind reminds your mind ... to pay more and more attention to that heaviness pulling down. And that arm can begin to move down now ... as that heaviness increases ... and it would be so comfortable just to allow that heavy arm to drift down now. That's right ... drifting down ... moving it down now ... letting it return to a comfortable resting position where it can relax completely ... and you can relax completely ... drifting down with it ... down into a deep deep trance ... as your arm relaxes and the mind relaxes as well ... and you drift deeper and deeper as I continue to talk ... and your hands and arms feel so comfortable ... comfortable and relaxed. That's right ... ...

Continue with session as planned.

The Garden (Deepener)

As you go deeper now ... your subconscious mind becomes open ... more accessible and receptive to new learnings ... to changing old beliefs ... as you relax so comfortably there ... just listening to the sound of my voice ... here ... so calm ... and a feeling of peace and tranquillity allows you to relax more and more ... with each easy breath ... with each gentle beat of your heart. As I count down from ten to one ... you can just let go and you can go deeper now ... with each count ... using each number to let go of stress and tension ... to go deeper now.

Ten ... As you allow each muscle and nerve in your body to relax ... letting go ... becoming calm ... you feel peaceful ... comfortable now. **Nine** ... Relax your mind and your body together ... and if you lose track of the progression of the numbers ... then that is fine ... just let go now ... as ... **Eight** ... You start to sense a gentle connection between your mind and your body ... and an inner wisdom. **Seven** ... Go deeper now ... and as you breathe out ... *(Start to pace with breathing)* ... start to breathe out fear ... breathing out anxiety now. **Six** ... letting fear ... anger and stress flow away from your body ... with every outward breath ... letting go now ... slowly ... comfortably ... calmly. **Five** ... And now with each outward breath ... I want you to start saying a word to yourself ... without moving your mouth or your tongue ... your breathing not changing ... your throat perfectly still ... on each outward breath ... say the word inwardly to yourself ... **calm** ... *(Pace with outward breath ... and repeat)* ... **calm** ... **Four** ... without thinking what it means ... without analysing the word ... just moving the sound inwards now ... so that it seems to come from an inner wisdom ... *(match breathing)* ... **calm** ... **Three** ... Gently now ... easily ... calmly ... calm ... letting go ... and whenever your mind strays from that sound ... and it will stray away ... then just acknowledge that fact and gently bring it back ... repeating to yourself the word ... **calm** ... *(Match breathing)* **Two** ... Continuing now to relax ... and to let go ... gently drifting down ... into peace and harmony of body ... mind ... and spirit ... **One** ... And as you continue to drift deeper still ... you begin to see ... sense or imagine yourself in a beautiful garden ... the sun is shining ... gently warming your skin ... comfortable ... You look across the lawn as it sweeps away to an ornamental pond ... with a fountain playing ... the water droplets sparkling ... glistening ... in the soft diffused light that filters down through the leaves and branches of the ancient trees that surround this garden ... shielding and sheltering this beautiful place. The grass is soft ... springy beneath your feet ... and as you walk ... you pass flower beds cut into the lawn ... filled with the most beautiful flowers and plants ... so many varieties and colours ... and you can be aware of the fragrance of the flowers carried to you on a soft breeze that drifts across the garden ... rustling the leaves ... causing the heads of the flowers to sway gently ... the subtle sounds of nature all around you ... birds singing ... the drone of insects and the splash and gurgle of cascading water ... each sound ... each sensation ... relaxing you more ... comforting as you drift deeper ... and every step becomes heavier.

You soon find yourself in a small clearing ... the sun warming you and relaxing you more and more now ... as you sit ... resting your back against a large and ancient tree ... the bark of the tree is soft and comfortable ... and you sense that many people have rested here as you are resting now ... and although you are alone ... you feel safe here ... peaceful ... comfortable ... the word **calm** ... comforts you more as your mind drifts and fades.

Continue with therapy session.

Cloud Deepener Relaxation

To achieve eye closure.

Now *(client's name)* ... I would like you to continue to allow that relaxation to deepen. You allow no tension at all to come into you ... You can allow your mind to clear totally of all worries and concerns ... and I want you to know that all forms of tension ... anxiety and depression that you may have had ... are all lifted from you and you will feel very very **relaxed** and calm within yourself.

Whenever you hear me say the word ... **relaxed** ... you will double your relaxation. You now experience complete peace and calm within yourself.

As you rest so quietly there ... **relaxed** ... and peaceful ... I want you to imagine that as you look upwards you can see the sky ... a clear blue sky ... with just one white fluffy cloud. And as you look at that one white fluffy cloud ... so it begins to descend ... getting lower and lower ... until it envelops you as you rest there. ... and that fluffy cloud seems to gently massage your body with soothing ... healing ... energy ... making you feel even more ... **relaxed**. ... You feel calm ... safe and secure ... You can feel the soothing energy gently massaging ... pulsating through the whole of your body ... in through the pores ... and flowing right through your body easing out any tensions ... depressions ... or anxieties ... out through your fingertips and your toes ... Any bad feelings ... any negativity ... all being pushed out. ... and this leaves you feeling so very calm ... so very **relaxed** .... so unconcerned.

If it is your wish ... as you recognise that you really are in control ... you may choose to allow your cloud to just drift upwards into the clear blue sky. ... And you can enjoy the wonderful clean ... pure fresh air ... or you may choose to float on your cloud ... surrounded by pure healthy energy ... and as you take a deep breath ... you can feel this healthy soothing energy flowing in through your nostrils ... all the way down your throat and into your lungs.

You can feel it enter your bloodstream ... and circulate to all parts of your body ... filling your very being ... soothing ... healing energy ... flowing all through your body ... You can feel your whole body tingle with pure ... healthy ... soothing energy.

Now take a deep breath ... and as you breathe out release finally any remaining negative emotions ... you feel so good now ... so in control ... so very comfortable as you continue now ... relaxing ... deeper and deeper.

Continue with therapy session.

Count Down Induction

To achieve eye closure.

And now that you are resting so quietly there with your eyes closed ... I am going to help you to relax even deeper ... I'm going to count ... very slowly ... up to seven ... and in between each count ... I'll use the words "drifting deeper and deeper". And you'll find ... as this count progresses ... that you can drift deeper into that trance state ... As I count you can help too as you tell yourself ... "I am going deeper and deeper into hypnosis".

Now it doesn't matter if your mind wanders ... It doesn't matter even if you lose awareness altogether ... All that matters now is your own relaxation ... so just be comfortable ... allow yourself the pleasure of sinking deeper and deeper into the comfortable cushion of that chair. Just let yourself drift into that relaxation as I count slowly up to seven ... using the words "drifting deeper and deeper" in between each count ... and I'll begin that count for you now.

One ... Drifting deeper and deeper ... **Two** ... Drifting deeper and deeper ... And already you can feel yourself settling down ... becoming much more relaxed now ... you're feeling so very comfortable ... beginning to feel peaceful too .... Just feel that relaxation ... working its way through your body. It's bringing every part of you to rest ... settling you right down.

Three ... Drifting deeper and deeper ... **Four** ... Drifting deeper and deeper ... And now you can be aware of how slow and easy your breathing has become ... a little slower and a little deeper too ... and each deep breath that you take is making you more comfortable and much more relaxed ... more and more relaxed ... just feel your whole body getting heavier ... comfortably heavier ... almost as though you're sinking down ... down ... just sinking down into sheer comfort ... as each breath you take ... relaxes you more ... and more ... and more.

Five ... Drifting deeper and deeper ... **Six** ... Drifting deeper and deeper ... You're feeling more comfortable ... more relaxed .... tired and so glad to be drifting deeper and deeper.

Heavy ... tired ... drifting deeper and deeper and relaxed. Beautifully relaxed. Every part of your body is coming to rest now. Feeling tired ... drifting deeper and deeper ... heavy and relaxed ... tired ... drifting deeper and deeper ... heavy and relaxed.

Seven ... Drifting deeper and deeper into that warm and comfortable state of just letting go completely ... allowing the subconscious mind to take on more and more of that responsibility for guiding your awareness ... down ... as you drift with your own thoughts ... just listening to the sound of my voice.

Each word that I speak now allows you to continue to drift now ... deeper and deeper into that relaxation ... nothing bothers you ... nothing disturbs you at all as you concentrate only on my voice ... Should the telephone ring ... it will not concern you ... Even the loudest of noises will not bother you at all as you listen to my voice ... concentrating only on the sound of my voice ... each word ... each sound relaxing you even deeper than before.

This is a special time for you ... a time to put aside all your worldly thoughts and material problems ... a time when you really can become aware of that inner part of you ... a time when no one is demanding anything from you ... no one needing anything from you. This is your time ... a wonderful relaxation of both your body and your mind.

Now *(client's name)* ... I am going to allow you just a short time of silence ... a few moments that you can use to settle down deeper into that comfortable state that you are enjoying right now ... using the ability that you have to drift even deeper into your own innermost mind. When I speak to you again ... in a few moments' time ... you'll be much more relaxed ... more comfortable ... feeling so safe and so secure ... far far more relaxed than you are now ... so just rest quietly now ... and enjoy the peace and the tranquillity of the next few moments ... until you hear my voice again.

(Allow about one minute)

Now as I slowly count down ... from five to one ... just let yourself drift deeper and deeper ... more and more ... into that relaxation *(Repeat)*. **Five** ... **four** ... **three** ... deeper and deeper ... drifting down and deeper still ... down and down .... **two** down ... down ... down ... down ... **one** (*Increase interval between counts)* Just rest and relax now. Just rest and relax.

Continue with therapy session.

The Stair (Deepener)

Now you can allow your inner mind to show you standing at the top of a fine marble staircase ... with ten steps leading down ... There is a firm handrail and here you feel safe and secure ... nothing concerns you at all ... and in a moment you can walk down that staircase and as you hear me count off each of the steps ... you can step down one step ... doubling your relaxation with each step that you take.

Begin now as I count ... **Ten** ... Doubling your relaxation ... going deeper (*Pace with breathing*) ... **Nine** ... Deeper still ... **Eight** ... Letting go of tension as you relax and go deeper. ... **Seven** ... Doubling your relaxation ... deeper still ... **Six** ... Aware now of your breathing and how comfortable it has become ... **Five** ... Each gentle breath relaxes you ... you relax more with each breath that you take ... **Four** ... Deeper ... even deeper into a state of profound relaxation of mind and body ... **Three** ... Doubling your relaxation going ever deeper ... **Two** ... The deeper you go the better you feel ... and you go deeper the better you feel ... **One** ... Almost all the way down now into total relaxation ... **Zero** ... Now stepping off the bottom step and you find yourself in a place that is comfortable and safe for you to be ... a place of safety and security where there is no anxiety ... no fear ... just tranquillity ... and calm peace.

Continue with session as planned.

Overload Induction

An induction for those clients who are extremely analytical, rigidly controlled.

Now I know how difficult it can seem to someone with your intelligence to recognise that it can make a pleasant change for me to have the privilege to work with someone of your intellectual ability ... instead of some who come **here** and sit in that relaxation chair **there** and even they ... with their eyes closed can be so small minded ... always appearing mad at the world and never giving a moment for themselves ... to relax ... Those are the ones who just feel that they have no need at all to listen to what is said or not said ... putting values on everything ... values that have no place ... **here** ... no value ... **there** ... as they refuse to learn anything that will help them to see the world in a different light ... that will allow them to care ... that they can care for themselves ... and be comfortable too ... It is so comforting too ... to know that you have that capacity to use your ability in that way ... to learn and to accept that it can be such a relaxing experience ... to allow that drifting into a trance to occur ... without concerning yourself ... as you try to be aware of all that is said ... the exact meaning of all the words ... and of all those events that occur in your own thoughts ... or awareness ... You can know too that you can choose ... to forget to choose to pay that attention to all that happens ... **here** in your experience or not ... **there** ... or what changes ... or stays the same ... and what about that man who set out to travel to a place where he needed to be? ... He knew that he had been told the right way to go ... keep to the left for the first part ... that's right ... so easy at first and then take that turn to the right ... that's right ... not the left because what is right is to take a right ... then what is left cannot be right until the turn that is next that is left ... the turn to the left that will be right that takes him straight to the next turn that is right ... and if that turn is right then he would be turning left onto the right road ... and then all that was left was to relax ... and be totally unconcerned ... because all that was left to do now was to continue ... right ... on down that road that went up the hill to the right of the white house on the left and then go right and then left ... to be absolutely right ... It really can seem to be too much effort at times to be so concerned about what is right ... that can best be left to those who need to know that which may turn out to be that ... or perhaps something else entirely ... which could be right too ... if that was all that was left ... And I know that you will be only too pleased to remember that ... when you consider that so many things can be the same but different too ... like one and one are two which can be also too ... and then two and two are four ... but then what for ... if not to relax and begin to recognise that you really do not know what is no **here** or yes **there** ... where to go ... to where you can let go and allow those things to occur in their own time ... as you let go while holding on to that new recognition ... that what you know is that which is ... that there is nothing that you require to do or not do as your ability allows you to be totally relaxed and comfortable ... as you recognise that what I say can mean so many different things ... It can be so easy to accept all those things and to be completely comfortable and relaxed with all that is so right ... and be left with that train of thought that could allow you to stay on track ... and recognise that too was not worth the effort ... that takes so much effort as you try to remember so many things ... and to understand **NO** need for understanding ... The conscious of your mind can do anything ... go any place it wishes to ... without that need at all for you to be so concerned that your subconscious is concerned ... to hear all that is important to you ... as you continue to listen to the sound of my voice that drifts down with you now ... into that calm drifting ... drifting of thoughts and of experience too ... that can go so slow so quickly now ... as that relaxation that is yours becomes more and more ... as you can allow the subconscious of your mind to take too ... the responsibility for guiding your thoughts and your experience into a quiet calmness that follows ... when dreams can be turning within ... as the wheel turns and the world turns ... all on its own ... nothing at all for you to do ... or to be concerned with at all as you drift effortlessly down into that drifting place where nothing is left ... but only what is right for you ... to where your own inner mind waits too with those wisdoms that are yours and those things needed too.

Continue with session.

Remembering Trance Experienced

Use with clients who have experienced trance before.

Now as you begin to make yourself so comfortable **there** ... I wonder if you can remember how easily you entered into that trance state before ... how good it felt to allow your eyes to close ... to concentrate on all of that tension ... becoming so aware and so in control of your own abilities to go into deep hypnosis ... just allowing that tension to flow away from you as every muscle relaxed ... every fibre relaxed ... as your mind relaxed too ... just letting go and drifting off as your own subconscious mind accepted the responsibility for guiding your awareness ... down ... deep into that comfortable heaviness of arms ... of legs ... of the whole body as you discovered that it can be so easy ... so pleasant ... to allow those feelings to continue ... to deepen even more as you listened to the sound of my voice speaking to you in soothing relaxing tones and to remember too that you really do have that ability ... to relax ... to let go completely and to be totally unconcerned that **there** is no need at all for you to be concerned about how much effort it takes ... to make an effort to try to hear ... or to understand everything that I say **here** or don't say **there** ... so much easier to just let go and allow all of those things to occur in their own time and in their own way ... and I know that you can co-operate with me so well ... that you can relax in that way ... drifting down to that place inside ... where all is still ... quiet ... peaceful ... where **there** is only the sound of my voice and the wisdom that is yours as you become more and more relaxed with that awareness of your own subconscious mind. Nothing bothers you ... Nothing concerns you ... as you continue to relax ... to go deeper than before ... each word that I speak relaxing you ... deeper ... deeper ... deeper.

As you continue now to allow your own subconscious to take on more and more of the responsibility for guiding ... for directing your awareness ... you can be aware too of the sound of my voice speaking to you as before ... **here** ... as you relax so completely ... **there** ... each word that I speak just a signal for you to relax ... to let go ... to drift even deeper now. You can be aware too of the sounds that surround you ... the sounds in the room ... ticking of the clock perhaps ... marking the passing of time ... time that can be so pleasant ... and even though so little time is needed the experience can be so enduring ... so much value to you ... and the subconscious can allow time ... time to be however long it is useful for you to experience ... when a short time can seem such a long time ... or a fleeting moment ... pleasurable moments ... comfortable and safe moments ... moments that combine now to continue ... as you enjoy that experience ... aware now even more than before of that inner part of you ... deep inside your own mind where all is truth and all is known ... every experience ... every part of you that makes you the unique personality that you are ... you in communion with you ... the you that is constant ... never tells you a lie ... gives you good advice ... speaking to you now **there** ... as I speak **here** ... And I wonder if you can allow that experience to continue now ... the same ... or to deepen even more as I continue to speak to you ... my words drifting ... as you drift now with your own thoughts ... thoughts that flit like butterflies ... a pleasant flash of colour ... and then gone ... drifting too into comfortable relaxation of mind ... relaxation of body ... heaviness of arms ... of legs ... of no concern to you now ... safe and secure ... **there** for you when you need them ... but for now they can rest ... relax ... relax ... in that comfortable place ... that haven deep inside ... my voice ... my words heard but not heard too ... Nothing bothers you or disturbs you as you continue now to utilise the power of your own subconscious inner mind to help you now with that problem ... that troublesome thing ... knowing that **here** within ... **there** you really do have the answer ... the solution ... so relax now ... and ask what you will ... to help you as I continue to speak to you....

Continue with therapy session.

Habit and Instinct

In order to develop strategies that will help others to modify behaviours which are described as 'habit', first we must begin with an understanding of the dynamics of habit formation.

A habit has been described as a learned response. Therefore any response that is developed through repetition can be described as habitual. Within this description we must therefore include skills. A carpenter becomes skilled in the use of his tools to the point where he really does not have to apply much in the way of conscious attention to the angle at which he holds a chisel or how he planes a piece of timber.

Through repetition he has developed a natural ability to carry out the tasks peculiar to his trade without the need to exercise the amount of conscious attention to detail that would be required of the amateur.

The response that occurs when a craftsman approaches a task is an habitual response, i.e. a response of the subconscious, not the conscious. But is that the same as the response which causes us to duck when a missile is thrown? I wonder sometimes just where do we draw the line that describes one response as habitual and another as instinctive?

If the habits that concern us, such as nailbiting, overeating, smoking or alcohol and drug abuse, are learned responses, then it must follow that they can be unlearned and that new responses to the stimulus can be introduced. The new responses introduced, if repeated, will eventually become the learned response to that stimulating factor or event and will therefore form a new habit.

Habits can be either desirable or undesirable, in the manner in which they affect our lives. The response to an event can either be adaptive or maladaptive according to the real effect. The smoker may feel that smoking is helping him/her because of the illusion of relaxation that is created when the discomfort that is the craving for nicotine is temporarily relieved by tobacco consumption.

The truth is that more harm than good is being done so what appears to be beneficial is in fact harmful and therefore can be described as maladaptive.

The approach that we take must be one that is constructed to take into account all of the variances that make up the habitual response. The subconscious will choose to justify the habit's continuance, so there is a necessity to understand the reason for the habitual response. Being convinced on a conscious level really will not do the trick alone.

'Reframing' is a technique that can be incorporated into the hypnotherapy approach, allowing the power of the client's own subconscious to change perception so that the new, adaptive responses being suggested will take effect. If we as therapists can facilitate implantation of new thinking that eases the sometimes impossible seeming conflicts that have hitherto sustained the unwanted habit, then we are well on the way to that repetition of desirable responses that will become the new and adaptive behaviour.

The scripts within this section contain many similarities simply because they are dealing with habits. Smoking, nail-biting and overeating constitute situations and events that create more harm than benefit, which can be addressed in similar ways.

Anchors

An anchor is simply a stimulus which initiates a response – for example, when you arrive in your dentist's waiting room you may experience anxiety or, when you see a police car in your rear view mirror, you may get a funny feeling and glance at the speedometer.

There is also a subconscious stimulus that results, for example, in the response of lighting up a cigarette – after a meal, on the telephone, with a drink, etc.

Of course the response can be a pleasant one such as the pleasure that we feel when we hear the voice of a loved one; a picture perhaps or a word that stimulates a warm glow of remembrance of a special event or person; the response that is experienced when a favourite treat is mentioned such as a Black Forest gateau. (But then that is my Achilles heel! I wonder, what is yours?)

These can be termed conditional responses, the stimulus being associated with a particular event or circumstance, but the important thing is that a response can be controlled to enable a particular event or stimulus to be linked to a desired response or reaction.

A stimulus can be any one of many occurrences, be it taste, feel, colour, hearing or smell. A most useful explanation is the following extract from *Neurolinguistic Programming, Vol 1:*

Anchoring is in many ways simply the user-oriented version of the stimulus response concept in behaviouristic models. There are however ... some major differences between the two. These include:

1) *Anchors do not need to be conditioned over long periods of time in order to be experienced. That kind of conditioning undoubtedly will contribute to the establishment of the anchor ... but it is often the initial experience that establishes the anchor most firmly. Anchors then promote the use of single trial learning.*

2) *The association between the anchor and the response need not be directly reinforced by any immediate outcome resulting from the association in order to be established. That is ... anchors or associations ... will become established without direct rewards or reinforcement for the association. Reinforcement ... like conditioning will contribute to the establishment of an anchor ... but is not required.*

3) *Internal experience (i.e ... cognitive behaviour) is considered to be as significant ... behaviourally ... as the overt measurable responses ... in other words NLP (Neuro-Linguistic Programming) asserts that an internal dialogue ... picture or feeling constitutes as much of a response as the salivation of Pavlov's dogs.*

(Dilts, Grinder, Bandler, Delozier, 1980)

Generic Habit Control

First induce hypnosis:

And now I would like you to allow your subconscious mind to allow you to see yourself standing at the top of a flight of steps ... I want you to be aware of how safe and comfortable you feel ... as you continue to listen to my voice ... and follow my simple instructions which are all for your benefit and well being.

As you allow your mind's inner eye to follow the flight of steps down ... you can become aware of the door at the bottom ... I would like you to tell me when you can see the door. (*Await response)* That's good ... You are doing very well ... I wonder if you can tell me what colour the door is? (*Await response)*

That's right ... the door is a colour that your subconscious knows is relaxing for you ... a colour that allows you to feel safe and secure ... Now I want you to begin to step down each step ... and as you step down each time I want you to say inwardly to yourself ... I am going deeper and deeper into hypnosis ... and then say out loud the number of that step as you descend from 10 all the way down to 1 ... relaxing deeper and deeper with every step ... with every breath that you take.

So begin now ... take your time ... and when you get to the bottom you will be even more deeply relaxed than you have been before ... When you reach the bottom you can tell me by just saying "I'm there". (*Wait for client to complete the sequence)*

That's so good ... you really are doing so well ... Now you are standing before that *(colour)* door ... Once again I want you to be aware of how safe and secure you are feeling. Nothing bothers you or disturbs you at all as you continue now to listen to my voice ... each word that I speak soothing and relaxing you even deeper now.

The door in front of you is the door to that part of your inner mind where all the very positive parts of you are centred ... All of your strengths and your determination to succeed are here ... All good feelings about yourself and recognition of yourself as a very special unique human being are here ... always ready to help you with any problem ... to give you the benefit of what is your own wise inner mind ... These are the parts of you that will always give you good counsel as they have only your best interests at heart ... These are those parts which make up what some call their own wise inner advisor ... that part that tells you the right thing to do ... Sometimes that part is so difficult to hear above the clamour and clatter of other considerations ... but today it will be speaking to you with total clarity as you now call upon it for the help that you need now.

Now see that door slowly opening ... and you can see within all of those parts ... welcoming you as you step forward into that comfortable room to join with all of your own positive personality ... Perhaps you can now sense that aura of well being here as you surround yourself with positivity ... determination ... courage and that powerful force that really is yours within.

Now I want you to look across the room ... to where in the back wall ... you can see another door ... This door is coloured the deepest black ... and I wonder whether you can see how large is the lock on that door keeping it securely closed.

Behind this door is another part of you ... a part that is not to be denied or underestimated. This is that part of you that continues to encourage you to indulge in *(habit or behaviour)* that you really do want to break away from.

This part hides away in that room so that it can do its worst ... locked away from those positive parts that could so easily destroy it so that it would never bother you again ... But now ... I am handing you the key to that lock and you can enter into the room beyond ... taking with you all of your powerful and positive forces of courage and determination to succeed ... confidence and self esteem ... knowing that combined now ... you can and you will confront that part and defeat its evil and destructive influence.

Now take the key and put it into the lock ... Notice how easily that lock opens as you with all your strength push the door open and enter into the room beyond to confront the part that is that habit. *(Describe habit or behaviour)*

Now you can see it there as it cowers in the corner ... terrified at the array of positive forces that you have with you now ... surrounding you in a cocoon of positive radiance ... Now with the help of your own inner mind and all of your positive forces ... you can tell that part that you want no more of it ... that it has no place in your life ... that you now banish it forever unless it agrees now ... to cease once and for all that destructive and sad behaviour and instead take on another role ... a more positive role ... that will be of use to you ... a role that you can choose for it right now ... Perhaps it can help you with your confidence ... or with your self esteem ... even your ability to be a better lover? Whatever you choose it must obey or be gone forever.

Now with all of your forces beside you ... you can ask that part if it is willing to do that which you are asking of it ... Do it now and tell me when you have that agreement. *(Await positive response. If there is any doubt, impress upon the client that this is his subconscious and that he is in control and must be obeyed.)*

Okay ... now you have that agreement ... and now that part is willing to join with those other positive elements of your unique and special personality ... so you can welcome it in ... Allow all those other parts of you to join with it and make a fuss of it as you and they lead it away from this place into the other room ... that place where only positive and beneficial elements can be ... that problem resolved and forgotten.

When you are satisfied that all is done that needed to be done ... then you can once again close and lock that black door sealing off that place where only negativity belongs ... and as you seal that door you seal behind it the memory of what was a problem before but is now no more ... Notice now that the door is changing colour ... no longer black and threatening for that power for bad is no more ... It is gone and forgotten.

Now, leaving your own inner mind more powerful and more dynamic than it was before, you can return now to wakeful awareness ... aware that you have all the confidence all of the determination and all of those good and beneficial thoughts about yourself that will sustain you and strengthen you in everything you do.

I will count from one to five and with each count you will drift back upwards bringing with you a feeling of strength and of self awareness of you as a stronger and more positive person ... a feeling that will grow stronger and stronger with every day.

One ... **two** ... **three** ... **four** ... eyes beginning to open and **five** ... eyes open and fully awake.

Guilt Trip

This is very effective when used at the beginning of the post hypnosis intervention. Please recognise that this approach can be used for so many maladaptive behaviours. Simply substituting the word 'smoking' with 'overeating', for example, will do the trick.

As you take a deep breath now ... I would like your subconscious to show you a room ... a familiar room perhaps ... Gathered here are all of those people who are special to you ... who love and care for you and whom you love and care for.

They have all come here today ... because you have something to explain to them all ... Your doctor has warned you that you must quit smoking because the next aneurysm/heart attack will more than probably prove fatal ... You will die an early death because you refuse to take responsibility for your own life and your own health ... For the sake of a noxious habit you are prepared to risk all ... In fact you have made a choice ... a choice to die an early death leaving behind all of these people who so much wish for you to give up that dreadful habit ... Now I want you to explain to all here why you choose to continue to smoke ... to risk with every cigarette that life that is so precious ... not just to you ... but to those here who rely on you to be there for them ... Go ahead and tell them why a cigarette means so much more to you than the love and care they give to you ... much more than the life that is so precious ... Tell them now the awful truth ... and watch their faces ... the dismay ... the horror ... the disgust ... the feelings of helplessness ... anger ... grief ... and how do you feel now? *(Await response and then continue with session)*

Snippet:

Small keys open large doors.

Nail Biting

Using Ideomotor response and anchors.

And now as you relax even deeper ... listening to the sound of my voice ... each word that I speak here can be a signal for you to go deeper still as you rest so comfortably and quietly there ... I wonder if you can really be aware now of how much more comfortable you can become ... as you begin now to sense in some safe and agreeable way ... a gentle connection between your mind and your body that has no part to play here ... all that is required is that you continue to allow those comfortable hypnotic sensations ... heaviness of arms ... of legs ... comfortably heavy ... to deepen even more ... as your whole body relaxes ... all tension just draining away ... and you can turn inwards now ... deep inside ... to where that part of you that is all knowing ... creative and perfect ... is ready now to do its best work for you ... to help you make those changes that you want to make ... that you can make and will make.

That's good *(client's name)* ... Now I would like you to allow your subconscious to take you back in time ... back to a time when you were really confident in your ability to take control and to be in control ... a memory of yours ... pleasant and reassuring ... when you really did feel good ... powerful ... assertive ... and allow that experience to develop and those good feelings to expand ... and when you are fully experiencing that event ... I want you to allow your subconscious to lift the index finger of your right hand ... *(Touch the finger – ideomotor response)* If you experience any difficulty in recalling a memory that is appropriate ... then that's fine ... you can allow your subconscious to create a scene where you are confident and in total control ... go ahead now ... *(Watch for responses including changes in skin tone and breathing as well as ideomotor response)*

(Now grasp firmly the shoulder or arm of the client and continue for about 10 to 15 seconds to establish the anchor)

That's good ... you are doing this very well ... and now I want you to allow that scene to fade and your mind to become calm and quiet as before. Now I would like you to allow your subconscious mind to show you a scene ... in the future ... at one of the next times when you bite your nails ... your hands staying where they are now comfortably in your lap there ... having no part to play here. ... Allow that scene and that experience to develop and become real ... those feelings to expand and grow ... and allow your subconscious to let me know when that is done ... as that index finger of your right hand can lift. *(Touch finger)*

(Watch for responses including changes in skin tone and breathing as well as ideomotor response. Now grasp firmly the shoulder or arm of the client as before and continue for about 10 to 15 seconds to "fire" the anchor.)

That's fine ... you really are doing this well ... and I wonder now just how you feel about biting your nails ... how you will find it so easy to not do that anymore ... remembering how unpleasant and how bad it made you feel because now you know what you are not going to do ... and how to remind yourself with an irresistible response ... reaching deep into the subconscious of your mind ... that you will never ever be able to do that again in that way or at all ... because if you do then you will be doing it on purpose ... and that's a different matter entirely ... it all belongs to you.

Trance termination.

Weight Loss Reframe

I would emphasise here that this reframing technique is universally adaptable and its applications are restricted only by the imagination of you the therapist.

I want you now to take a deep breath ... and then as you breathe out you will go ten times deeper into relaxation ... and you can concentrate fully on that thing which is so important ... that habit of overeating ... eating unhealthy and fattening foods ... something that you really do want to change ... but there is something stopping you.

As you allow that relaxation to deepen even further ... you will be aware of when I say the word 'now' ... When you hear that word you will relax ... doubling your hypnosis each time.

Now I know that changing that overeating habit really is important to you ... I would also like you to know that what I have so often found ... is ... that there is an unconscious part of you that is preventing you from making those changes.

Now if that is the case here ... now ... I would like to ask that part of you ... to come forward and make itself known, to you in some safe way that you can understand ... so please ... *(client's name)* ... go deep inside now into your own inner mind ... wherever you need to go to become aware of that part of you that is responsible for this habit of overeating.

Now it is difficult for me to know how you will experience that part of you that is responsible for your overeating ... it may be a familiar experience or one that is unique to you ... something that you see in your mind's eye ... perhaps a picture ... a face ... or a scene ... It could be any visual image ... or perhaps it may make itself known to you as a voice or a sound ... it could be your own voice or that of another ... or perhaps you will experience it as a feeling or emotion of some kind ... so as you go into your inner mind ... I am asking with respect that that part that is responsible for this overeating habit ... allows itself to be made known to you in some safe way.

Now *(client's name)* tell me, are you experiencing anything that could be that part now allowing you to be aware of it ?

(If no experience is reported, continue): That's fine ... your unconscious may not be happy with your experiencing in that way ... but please proceed with the understanding that your subconscious will understand and will co-operate with us here today.

(Experience reported, continue): That's good ... now allow that experience to grow and expand so that you are sure of that communication. I would like to thank that part for coming forward and suggest that you do too.

I would like you to know that the part of you that is responsible for your overeating ... deserves respect ... It is obviously very powerful because even though you have wanted to make this change ... you haven't been able to do so. I also understand that this part of you that is responsible for your overeating habit will change only when it is ready to do so.

I want to suggest to you *(client's name)* that in some way ... overeating has in the past ... provided some benefits and has been useful to you ... in the past ... that in some way you have gained an advantage ... Okay, I fully understand that the experience of the behaviour of that part responsible for your overeating has been the cause of negative and unhealthy consequences for you ... but what I am suggesting is that you now re-examine your understanding of the intention of that part and accept that is has been doing this in order to help you and to benefit you in some way. Now take some time to go into your own inner mind and become aware of just what the benefits and advantages have been for you ... Perhaps that part has been helping you to avoid something that is unpleasant or painful ... or helped you get something that you desired ...

Or perhaps it has helped you in providing a relief or substitute for something that is missing from your life ... perhaps the love that you need ...

Or perhaps the confidence that you need to achieve what you want.

There is a tendency to associate fat people with being slow ... lazy ... unintelligent ... and so being fat can be an excuse for not trying ... It is not expected and so the pressure is relieved.

Or, "Men will not be able to hurt me if I am unattractive ... they will leave me alone."

Your unconscious ... that part of you will allow you to know now the truth and how it has done what it has done to help you.

I am asking you again *(client's name)* to assume that the part of you responsible for your overeating has continued up to now ... because it has helped you or benefited you in some way ... so please become aware now ... if it is comfortable and safe to do so ... of just how this overeating habit has helped you in the past.

Now keeping those benefits ... or perhaps we can call them pay-offs ... in mind ... I would like to suggest to your subconscious that there are alternative patterns of behaviour ... of experiencing ... of perception ... that can provide for you those benefits and pay-offs provided in the past by overeating ... but that can be much healthier and more satisfying for you and allow you to be happier ... So now that you have constructed patterns of behaviour and of perception which are more beneficial and yet still provide you with the benefits which are important to you ... now I want you once again to go deep inside to your subconscious and ask if there is any part of you which objects to these new arrangements that will allow you to eat correctly the right foods in the right amounts and achieve that slim and healthy body that you deserve.

Go ahead now ... and allow me to know the answer ... Are there any objections to these new alternative patterns of behaviour? ... Yes or no.

(If there are no objections, continue):

Okay that's good ... You have constructed for yourself new and beneficial patterns of behaviour that will allow your subconscious to help you with positive habit-forming affirmations to ensure that you achieve all of your worthwhile goals. I suggest that you now thank your subconscious for its co-operation and that you consciously work with it towards your goal.

Enuresis in Children

Direct approach with reframe.

Have the child bring along a favourite toy such as a doll or teddy bear that they would normally take to bed with them.

Hello *(client's name)* ... do you know why Mummy has brought you to see me today? Well, what we are going to do is play a little game that I know ... would you like that?

I see that you have brought *(teddy or dolly)* along to see me ... would you tell me his/her name? I bet you play with him/her a lot, don't you? ... and I bet too that you are very good at pretending, aren't you? ... Would you like to play a game of pretend with me now ? Good, its very very easy to play ... all you have to do is just sit there as still as you can and then close your eyes for me ... Can you do that? ... Mummy is going to play as well and she is going to close her eyes as well ... and I want you to pretend just as hard as you can ... that you just can't open your eyes at all ... and you can pretend so very hard that even if you want to open them you just can't ... and when I want you to open your eyes ... you won't be able to until I say special magic words ... When I say, "Teddy says open your eyes", then you will be able to open your eyes ... but if I don't use those magic words then your eyes will shut tighter and tighter until I say, "Teddy says open your eyes" ... and that's because you are pretending so well ... better than anyone else can ... That's very good.

Now as I talk to you about something very important, you can hear all of my words but they all help you to pretend even harder than before that your eyes just will not open until I say the magic words ... and you can feel so nice and comfy sitting there in my comfortable magic chair ... Nothing worries you at all ... and perhaps you can notice that you feel a little sleepy ... just a little bit ... so cozy there ... so warm ... cuddling teddy now ... and as I talk to you you can think about something very important to you ... It's about that little problem that you have been having when you go to sleep in your cozy bed ... that you are so cozy and warm that you sometimes forget to remember that you need to wake up when you need to wee wee ... You just forget to wake up and you have an accident that makes you feel so sad ... and then Mummy has to come along and change all of your bedclothes because they are all wet and uncomfortable for you ... and you really do want to remember not to forget to remember when its so important ... don't you? ... I know that you think it would be so much better to remember not to forget ... and remember when you need to wake up and go to the toilet ... and you wouldn't even need to wake Mummy ... Wouldn't it be good if you could do that every time?

Now I think that you could need just a little help from a very good friend of mine who helped me when I was a little boy, to learn how to remember how to not forget to wake up in time ... and he has come here today to help you too ... he is going to show teddy just how to help you remember every time that you need to go to wee wee ... and do you know ... he's so good at this ... you can be sure that you will never ever have that problem ever again. My friend's name is Tommy Tinkle and he comes from a long way away ... where all of the fairies and the elves and the gnomes come from ... It's a place where all of the magic in the world comes from ... somewhere very very special. Tommy is five hundred and two years old ... and he even knows Santa Claus ... he helps him at Christmas to make sure that all the children in the world get their presents on time ... He works very hard.

In a moment I'm going to call Tommy and he has promised me that he will come here by magic to see you today ... All I have to do is to say, "Tommy Tinkle from over the moon grant my wish and be here soon", and he will come right away ... but only you and I will be able to see him ... and only while our eyes are shut tight ... I am going to call him now, "Tommy Tinkle from over the moon grant my wish and be here soon". My, that was quick ... He is here already and as you are pretending so well you can see him sitting in front of you on a little stool. He is funny looking, only as big as teddy, and just look at what he has on ... a little red jacket with lots of silver buttons ... bright green trousers ... and yellow shoes with big buckles on the toes ... and what a funny pointed hat ... He even has a curly feather in it ... and he looks so very happy ... always laughing because he likes children very much. ... I wonder if you can count the buttons on his jacket ... How many are there? ... That's very good ... Now *(name)* say hello to Tommy ... and I will tell you what he is going to do ... that he did for me when I was a little boy and found it so hard to remember to wake up in time to go to wee wee in the toilet ... A friend of my Mummy's asked Tommy Tinkle to come along and help me to remember to wake up in time ... You see I had a teddy just like yours ... and Tommy showed my teddy just what to do and gave him some magic so that he would know just when I needed to wake up ... to go to the toilet ... to wee wee ... and I never ever had a nasty wet bed ever again ... I was so pleased and my Mummy was pleased too because she never had to get up to change those wet sheets ever again ... Now he's going to do that for you ... and he is going to come over there and whisper in teddy's ear the magic words that will help him to make sure that you always remember ... because teddies never ever forget magic words. He will be very careful as he climbs onto the chair beside you ... so that he can whisper in teddy's ear ... It won't take very long now ... so that teddy will know exactly what to do for you ... Have you finished now Tommy? ... That's good ... He's nodding to me because I can't hear him like teddy can ... Perhaps you can hear him ... I know that when I was little I could hear him, but now that I am grown up I can't ... because only children can talk to elves and hear what they say.

Now teddy is going to show you what he has learned ... He knows exactly what to do ... and what to say to help you when you need to wee wee in the night ... but you must remember always to take him to bed with you ... and I know that Mummy will remember too ... Teddy is showing you now what he is going to do to wake you up ... What's he doing to you *(name)? (Wait for response, such as "he is pulling my hair ... or tugging my nose ... shouting in my ear")* That's wonderful ... That's exactly what my teddy did to me.

Now Tommy has to talk to a very special part of you deep inside your mind ... he is going to tell that part of you that has forgotten to tell you to get up to go to wee wee that it can help you now to do things in a much different way that is so much better for you ... And I wonder of you can help too by asking that part to tell you why it has not woken you up in time before ... and then ask it if it can make sure that you have the same things as it was trying to give you before, but now, at the same time as helping you, also remembering to wake you up to go to the toilet .... Can you do that? *(wait for positive response)* That's so good ... you have done so very well.

Now Tommy has to go because he is very very busy ... so say thank you to him and good-bye now. "Good-bye Tommy".

Now teddy knows what to do ... and what to say ... He has all the magic to help you never ever to forget ... Now you can take him home ... and you will always remember to take him to bed with you every night, then he will be there to wake you when you need to wee wee and you will never ever have a nasty wet bed ever again ... so you will remember ... won't you?

You have been so very good at pretending and playing this little game with me, that Tommy has asked me to tell you that he is going to speak to Santa Claus and tell him just how good you have been ... and he is going to tell the tooth fairy to leave you something very special when she comes to see you. Now I am going to say those magic words so that you can open your eyes and be very happy and proud at being so clever at pretending here with me today. "Teddy says open your eyes".

Blowaway Technique

Ask the parent or guardian if they would like to participate in the session.

Take the child into hypnosis.

Now while everybody is nice and relaxed ... I want you *(child's name)* to cast your memory back into the years that have gone ... back into your growing up years ... I want you to think back to that first day at school ... You will remember that there were lots of emotions ... some very upsetting ... Think of how horrible it is to feel really sad ... and choked up with tears ... Think how awful it is to feel ashamed ... really ashamed. Think of how it is to feel anger ... fear ... feeling terribly small ... feeling alone ... imagining all kinds of things ... "

A lot of these things that you have been thinking about are bound to be upsetting ... so I want you to go to the **most upsetting** thing in your life ... the thing that frightened you the most ... or even the thing that embarrassed you the most ... as you are sitting there so nice and relaxed ... just think about it now ... and as soon as you have just thought about it ... so blowwww it away ... get rid of it now ... phwwwooo ... blowww it away ... phwwwoo ... blowww it away ... phwwwoo ...

If the child is really upset, move over to him or her and say, "Now stay still ... just stay still ... I want you to say three or four words about what is upsetting you ... just three or four words about that one thing that is really upsetting you ... Tell me what it is ... ?

"That's all done with now ... That's all over with now ... You can leave it all behind ... It used to be upsetting ... Now it's all right ... Come right up to date ... Start thinking about today ... It's all right now ... Think of all the nice things ... because when we finish here today you will feel much much better ... more confident ... you'll feel much more relaxed ... you'll find all those things that used to worry you ... they are gone now ... they are all gone now ... now you will find that instead you feel much more confident at school ... It's good to go back there ... you'll enjoy it ... you'll like seeing your friends ... You'll amaze yourself how much you are going to enjoy going to school ... Now in your own mind ... I want you to count up to five and when you reach five ... just open your eyes please."

If necessary give the child a protective bubble.
Attributed to Auriole Hitchcock FIAH.

Anxiety States

Phobias and fears are what bring so many clients to see a therapist. These clients require from therapists a special kind of understanding, because the fears that are blighting their lives so often appear inexplicable to the rational mind.

What is a phobia if it is not an irrational fear? The fear, the sheer panic, that is the experience of the sufferer is so real and the emotional pain so intense that it would be a complete affront to his dignity or self-esteem to tell him to get a grip on himself.

We need to gain an insight into the manner in which the subconscious interacts with sensory input which provides us with our perception of the world. We also need to understand how our belief system provides restraints upon our perception.

Throughout our life we are constantly updating the store of knowledge that helps us to identify objects, sounds and sensations. We begin with a pre-programmed set of instincts that can be best illustrated by considering the feeding impulse and the fright response in a baby. As time and experience provide more and more information to be assimilated, we become better equipped and better able to search and find stored data that is pertinent to the stimuli that is delivered through one or more of our senses.

As we grow older the mass of information stored in our memory continues to increase, so each search for pertinent information has more and more to draw upon. There comes a point when the smallest of clues can be enough to enable the subconscious to provide enormous quantities of information that relate to the experience.

Consider for example a situation where you are sitting in your lounge and you hear the sound of water filling the bath upstairs. Immediately you have a picture of the bathroom and all of its furnishings – the colour of the tiles around the bath, the picture on the wall, the sound of water gushing in the bath – all created within your imagination from information that has been stored.

The picture that is painted is the product of your imagination – your perception of that room and its function. If the wallpaper or floor covering or any other aspect of that room had been changed since you last formed your perception, then it would no longer be accurate.

To take the scenario one step further, we can consider the person who has in early life had a bad experience with a dog. The perception that has been formed regarding the dog is of something extremely unpleasant – with large teeth and a propensity to bite. Each time a clue is interpreted as 'dog', then the information that is available within subconscious memory is delivered up to complete the picture of 'dog'. That is then that person's perception of 'dog'. The whole picture is one that promotes anxiety and the invocation of the flight or fight response – rapid breathing, heart beating faster, adrenaline production as the body prepares itself to either run from danger or fight.

The reason for the fear in this case is not so far removed from what we can consider a logical reaction to meeting with a dog, as it can be explained in terms of actual experience. The reaction to the dog however becomes just a bit other than logical when it invokes a panic response at even the thought of a dog and when there has been plenty of opportunity through experience to gain a more realistic perception of dogs in general.

At a conscious level the subject knows that the dog is not vicious and that other people around can have a fun relationship with the animal in perfect safety, but nevertheless their reaction is that of panic beyond all reason.

We have to look further for our explanation of what is happening at a subconscious level and divorce ourselves from the application of pure logic to the situation.

So, what could be happening here? The subconscious has an ability to repress memories that are unpleasant and so spare us from the constant reliving of a particular event. A memory can be buried deep within the subconscious where it is beyond the reach of conscious recall, but buried with it are the anxieties and emotions attached to that event and these can hubble and bubble within seeking some way of manifestation. These are the feelings that Freud describes as 'free floating anxieties' ... anxieties that cannot be attributed to any event or object and which can be described so often as 'panic attacks'.

The subconscious finds a way to help us to deal with the anxieties, but first the anxiety must be turned into fear, and to fear it is necessary to have a focus. The actual memory of the event is repressed and buried beyond recall, so now the subconscious will play a trick and provide a substitute, something to which the anxiety can be attributed. Through avoidance of that chosen focus the fear situation is addressed. Why else would anyone have reason to fear a mouse or a spider which have so much more to fear from us than we have from them?

The solution in this case is to use hypnosis and regression techniques to go right back to the causative event, the memory of which exists deep within the subconscious. If we can bring to conscious attention the actual event then this presents us with a wonderful opportunity to form a new perception of that event which is positive and thus overcome the phobia.

The phobia just goes away, and the inappropriate and maladaptive mechanism for coping, which is the phobic irrational fear, is redundant. It sounds like magic, and, when it happens, the release of emotion can appear so powerful and so life-changing, that 'magical' is okay!

We may conclude that the world as we know it is predominantly a product of our own imagination. What we actually see or hear, touch or smell, plays just a minor role, as the slightest sensual stimulus provokes our subconscious to fill in much of the detail. Thus each of us, in our unique and individual way, arrives at what we believe is real.

Panic Attack

First of all I want you to remember a time when you felt happy and at peace with yourself ... when you felt safe and secure ... When you have done this just say 'yes'.

If you cannot remember a time when you felt happy ... secure and safe ... create a scene in your imagination where you can be totally safe ... happy and secure ... and perhaps you can have someone there with you ... some special person whom you feel safe with ... someone you can rely on to be protective and strong for you.

In future ... you will keep with you a notebook and pen ... You keep these with you so that you can write down all the thoughts ... all the symptoms and the emotions ... that you experience during a panic attack.

If you suffer from a panic attack you will recognise the absolute truth ... that no one has ever died from a panic attack ... You will concentrate on all the physical symptoms you are experiencing ... sweating ... palpitations ... trembling ... feeling nauseous ... the hot flushes ... and then write down all the thoughts ... the emotions ... that flash through your mind ...

Soon there will come a time when you are ready ... but in no more than seven days from today ... when you will accept my suggestion and learn to look forward ... to anticipate your panic attacks ... When you awake in seven days' time ... you will have learned to look forward to your panic attack as an experience ... because you will recognise that if you are looking forward to that panic attack ... it can no longer hold any fear for you ... you will no longer be afraid of a panic attack.

You already know now that you have that ability and that knowledge to relax yourself ... you know how you can take those ten deep breaths ... and then relax yourself completely ... letting go of tension and anxiety ... as you accept that new image of you ... there now ... feeling completely at ease ... safe and secure ... happy and at peace with yourself and your world ... You are in control ... and with each new day that feeling of control will grow and expand ... and you will be much more calm ... more relaxed ... your own person.

Soon there will come a time when you are ready ... but in no more than seven weeks from today ... you will deliberately try to invoke a panic attack ... In seven weeks' time ... you will try as hard as you can to bring about a panic attack ... a self-induced panic attack ... and you will concentrate on all those thoughts and all those symptoms ... that experience of having a panic attack ... and you will concentrate on building those experiences into a full blown panic attack.

When you have done this successfully ... and you can do it whenever you want to experience a panic attack ... then you can have a panic attack every night ... just one every night for a week ... Then you will get one of your own free will ... just once a week ... and then once a month ... and as you do this you will find that you will no longer suffer from panic attacks ... because you will be in control .... You will have learned that if you can have a panic attack when you want to ... then it is because you are controlling them ... They come only when you want them too ... and that is the strange and comforting truth ... **You have no need to have them at all** ... Yours is the choice ... is it not?

(Await response)

Trance termination.

Snippet:

Every opinion has a value – the value that you place upon it.

Strategy for a Past Life Recall (P.L.R.)

Before embarking on a past life recall, I explain carefully to the client the powers of the imagination and the nature of memory. It is important that the client is aware of the possibility that memories recalled may be simply those of watching a film or reading a book or are even just an imagined event. The subconscious memory does not differentiate and will accept all memory as actuality. What the client chooses to accept as truth must be left entirely to them. Whether or not you the therapist accept or deny the truth of the events occurring is of no consequence.

Carry out a lengthy induction.

Deepening with imagery:

Now I would like you to imagine yourself in a place that will provide for you feelings of peace and comfort ... security ... tranquillity ... It may be winter ... summer ... spring or autumn ... There may be trees ... mountains ... water ... lush green meadows ... or perhaps a beach with the waves rolling in from the ocean ... whichever place you choose is a place of peace and harmony and you feel totally safe and secure here ... and as you become more and more involved with this place that you have chosen you can relax even deeper than before ... relaxing ... releasing ... just letting go completely.

This is your own private and secret place ... and you are aware that this place is your own haven deep inside where only peace and harmony abide ... and you can go so much deeper now ... turning inwards to your innermost self ... where all knowledge and all memories are kept safe for you ... some easily accessible ... others hidden deep where they cannot be so easily recalled ... but they are there ... each and every one ... never forgotten ... from so far back in this life and from a time when this life was not yet begun ... memories that have shaped and moulded your unique and special personality ... and as you go deep inside now ... you can begin to experience a gentle connection with that special part of you that holds those memories that you now wish to explore and to re-experience ... That part now makes itself known to you in some special and safe way that you can recognise easily ... tell me *(client's name)* do you have any special or strange feelings or sensations? *(Wait for response. When your client reports any strange or unusual sensation, sound or image, continue)*

Okay, that's good ... Now let that feeling or experience grow stronger as you go deeper inside to connect more fully with that part of you. Now I am going to speak direct to your subconscious mind and I am going to ask your subconscious for permission to conduct a past life recall ... I want your subconscious to give me the answer ... Please do not do anything at all ... just continue to enjoy the peace and comfort of this place that you have chosen.

(The use of ideomotor response can be utilised at this juncture)

I am now going to touch your forehead and ask the question ... my words go direct into your subconscious and the answer ... either 'yes' or 'no' ... will come direct from that part of you ... Please do not involve yourself at all as your subconscious mind provides the answer to my question. *(Touch centre of forehead with finger)*

Am I speaking to that part of *(client's name)* which is able to give me permission to conduct a past life recall? ... Please answer 'yes' or 'no' ... *(Wait for response. If answer is 'yes' you can proceed)* Thank you, subconscious mind, for communicating with me ... I have been asked by *(name)* to help him to go back to that time before this current life to a previous existence ... Do I have your permission to do this and help in this way ? Answer 'yes' or 'no'. *(Await response. If response is 'yes', then continue)*

Thank you, subconscious mind ... I know that you will be there to ensure that all that is revealed will be done in a manner that is safe and beneficial for *(client's name).*

(Remove finger from forehead)

Now *(client's name)* we can proceed but first ... for your protection ... I want you now to see forming around you ... a white light ... a warm and comforting glow that surrounds you and envelops you in its protective aura ... a safe protective cocoon that will remain with you throughout the coming experience and beyond. Know now that I am with you at all times and that at any time ... if I touch you on the shoulder like this *(Touch shoulder with a firm but gentle pressure)* ... you can then immediately safely return to this time and this place ... here ... now ... to safety and peace and nothing can harm you or disturb you at all.

Now I am going to count to three and then snap my fingers ... and you will find yourself with me in a long corridor that stretches back through time ... right back through to the beginning of this life. You will see that there are many doors on either side of the corridor and behind each of these doors are stored memories of this life ... some good, some bad and also others that your subconscious mind has kept from you ... and as you walk along the corridor ... as you pass each of these doors ... you will be aware of feelings and emotions ... images ... sounds and experiences that emanate from within each of the rooms behind each of these doors. It may be that behind one of these doors is a memory that has been causing you pain in this life ... a memory of an event that needs to be addressed here and now ... Your subconscious mind will guide you here ... and should there be a particular door which merits your attention ... you will be drawn to this door ... and you will know that before we proceed further ... this door must be opened and you must deal with what lies within that room beyond. So go ahead now ... walk along that corridor ... past each of these doors ... Ahead of you at the end of the corridor you can see in the distance a door ... so much heavier ... so much more imposing than all of these along the sides ... This door is that door through which you passed into this life from beyond ... and it is this door that you must now go through to see what was before ... and it awaits you now ... You have the key and it will open for you ... but you must pass by all the other doors of this life before you can pass through this one. Go ahead now ... Take your time ... If there is a door that beckons you before you reach this special door ... then that is okay and we can pause to deal with whatever needs to be done ... You can speak to me clearly now as we go ahead ... but you cannot wake ... Just tell me when you are at the door to that life before ... or a door that needs to be opened here before we go on ... I am with you at all times.

(Events as they occur will determine progress. It may well be the case that the client will be compelled to enter a door on this side of the veil. Here you should proceed ... allowing him to enter that room and deal with the content which may be the cause of some problems in this life. Proceed down the corridor when the client feels able to leave that room ... into the corridor ... and then firmly close the door on the memory accessed ... having dealt with it in an appropriate and beneficial way. You as the therapist must use your best judgement.)

Now as you stand before that door that all those years ago you entered through into this life ... are you now certain that you wish to open that door and step through to whatever lies beyond? *(Await response)*

Okay ... that's fine ... I want you now to see the key to that door in the lock ... Reach out now and turn that key ... Feel it turn easily ... Now push open that door. Now I will count to three and on the count of three you will find yourself in a time before this time ... this life ... in a place where you have been in another time ... where you have lived before. **One** ... **two** ... **three**. Where are you now? ... Are you inside a building or outside? How old are you? ... What is your name? ...

(The questions that you ask are of necessity in accordance with the natural progression of the client's experience. The main points at this stage are to ascertain details of age, sex, nationality and profession, questions as to family and friends, etc., to determine the period in which this life was lived. I remember many years ago being advised to allow my own subconscious to help me, and I should like to pass on this suggestion. I personally record the sessions in order that facts that arise can be checked by the client if that is his or her wish.)

(At the end of every life there is a death, and this is a matter which can be important to the client's experience. Obviously there can be violence, sometimes horrific events, but you have assured your client that they are beyond harm. Remember to use the name that is given in the life recalled when speaking to your client.)

Now *(client's name!)* in a moment I am going to count from one to three and then I will snap my fingers ... and you will find yourself in that time ... in that place ... just before you pass into spirit. **One, two, three, "snap"**. Please tell me where you are and what is happening to you.

(Here you will be exploring the circumstances of death. It could be sickness, violence or just old age. The client may have died alone or with others around. Your questions will elicit the details.)

Now when I snap my fingers you will leave this life ... passing into spirit. **"Snap"**.

Now let's go to your funeral ... Who is there? ... What does it say on your memorial? etc. etc. ...

When I snap my fingers again ... I want you to find yourself in that place where all souls go between lives ... **"Snap"**. Describe to me now this place where you are ... Are there any people in the life that you have recalled that are there with you now? Are there any people there who will be with you in your next life?

What was the purpose of the life that you have just recalled? ... Were you successful in that life ... achieving that purpose?

Now as I count from one to five ... I want you to find your way back to that door through which you came to this life recalled ... Now go through that door into the corridor and then firmly close the door behind you and turn the key.

Now I want you to return to the place of comfort and safety where you were before we began the recall ... Relax now and enjoy the peace and calm tranquillity of this place ... Notice now that the white light that enveloped you ... is still with you ... all around you ... a protective aura ... and as you relax deeper now ... that white light begins to enter into your body to be absorbed ... to become part of you and you can feel its positive force ... its comforting energy ... as it circulates within your body now ... relaxing you ... calming you ... You feel an emotional calm that cancels out any unpleasant feelings and emotions that you may have had and you feel more relaxed and comfortable than you have ever felt before.

In a few moments ... you will be able to return to full conscious awareness. You will remember everything that is safe and beneficial for you to remember about your previous life recalled ... Your experience will strengthen you and help you to better accept those things in life which will remain forever unclear ... and you will be aware of feelings of peace and calm ... a gentle acceptance of what is to be ... allowing you now to feel free of anxiety about what will be ... as that new understanding deep within your subconscious is utilised to your highest benefit.

Trance termination.

Past and Interlife Experience

For use in past life and interlife regression sessions

Now as you relax so very comfortably there and begin to travel into a state of deep relaxation ... breathing easily and deeply now with your eyes closed listening to my voice and beginning now to enjoy the experience of deep relaxation as it overwhelms you now ... each word that I speak helps you to relax even more as you proceed ... slowly at first before you take that step that will lead to that celestial sanctum ... moving inside now deep within yourself ... moving steadily ... focusing on moving deeper and deeper into an altered state of that which appears real. Nothing concerns you at all except your own mind and the sound of my words as you go deeper with your consciousness.

Moving ever deeper ... please visualise now high above ... far beyond the clouds in the sky ... a huge and ancient building ... and know that this magnificent and beautiful place ... is a holy place ... much larger and much grander than any holy place of worship that could be found here on earth ... This celestial sanctum has a colossal double doorway ... beneath huge arches and massive towering twin spires.

Leading to the massive entrance is a set of huge stone steps ... Concentrate on bringing into being this vast holy sanctum ... every minute detail of its elaborate masonry ... and then see yourself poised at the foot of the steps looking up expectantly at the doorway ... Now start climbing the steps ... and notice the rough hewn granite as your shoes touch each step ... one after the other ... It's a long long climb ... but at last you reach the top and stand beneath the immense wooden door. Breathe deeply ... Pause ... Now stretch out a hand to feel the rough texture of the wood ... Brush your hand lightly over the varnished surface ... Feel the cracks ... the knots ... the joins in the heavy timbers. Now give a slight push to one of the doors and notice how easily it swings slowly open ... inviting ... as gradually the dimly lit interior is revealed and you step inside across the threshold onto the echoing flagstones of the vestibule.

Stand there now and look around you ... Observe the high vaulted ceilings ... the stained glass windows ... the massive columns and row after row of wooden benches. Shafts of light slant diagonally across these benches ... the air smells sweetly of incense and you are overwhelmed by the solemnity ... the stillness and the magnificence of the scene. Rather than proceed down the main aisle towards the great altar ... you turn instead to the left and walk towards the far wall. It's a long way away. As you walk be aware that the flagstones beneath your feet have given way to a floor of polished marble and that the wall is panelled in dark hardwood from floor to ceiling. Now look along that wall for a door ... a small door ... It's not easy to see ... You must look carefully. But at last you observe a small brass door handle and you proceed towards it. When you get there ... open that door ... and when you walk through that door ... you see a stone stairway. The steps are worn and narrow ... and they lead down into the cellars ... Move down these steps ... Feel yourself descending deeper and deeper into the very foundations of the building. At the foot of the stairway stands a man ... an old man. His hair is white and he is wearing a long black gown that reaches almost to his ankles. He is the guardian of the records and he is expecting you here ... but he wants to know why you are here. Explain your quest for self exploration and ask to see the record of your last inter-life. The old man ... bowing his head … listens attentively to your explanation and grants your request.

Next your guardian beckons you to follow him into the library. You seem to float behind the flapping hem of his gown as he sets off through the seemingly endless corridors ... past shelf after shelf piled high with books and video cassettes.

At last he comes to a halt between parallel lines of stacked volumes. He stands there for a few moments before pointing to a particular shelf of books and video cassettes ... You follow the line of his arm ... and your gaze alights upon your own name inscribed on the shelf in gold embossed lettering. Read this name and verify that it is indeed the name by which you are known ... then survey the books and video cassettes that are on the shelf ... your shelf.

There are many ... many books many … many video cassettes on this shelf of yours ... one for each of your past lives and one for each of your interlives. Observe the succession of leather spines ... placed in chronological order from left to right. As this life is not over yet and its record has not been completed ... the book and video cassettes on the extreme right are those that contain the record of your most recent interlife experience. Ask the guardian for this record and watch him steadily as he reaches up and retrieves the book or video that is applicable … and hands it to you. Hold the volume firmly ... feeling the texture of its soft leather cover ... and know that in a few moments you will open its pages to observe the contents of your last discarnate experience. If you have been handed a video cassette then you may use the video player that is there for that purpose. You may choose to look at any aspect of the interlife ... the threshold ... the judgement board ... planning the next life ... anything you wish. When you open the book or view the video ... you will see or hear with no fear ... words ... pictures ... even events that appear to you as they occurred ... moving pictures ... sounds ... experiences. What is contained therein has already happened … It presents no surprises to your subconscious ... You are merely looking at the record.

Now ... open the book or move the video forward or back and examine whatever section you have selected. Absorb the record calmly ... passively ... without emotion. You have all the time that you wish.

When you have seen all that there is to see ... close the book or switch off the video player and hand back either the book or cassette to the guardian who is waiting patiently some distance away. He replaces the book or video cassette on its shelf and then motions for you to follow him once more through the labyrinthine corridors to the stairway leading back to the great hall. You hasten after the old man until you are brought to the place where you first met. There you bid him farewell for the time being and ascend the stairs ... proceeding back to the silence and majesty of the great hall. You close the door behind you and pause for a moment to savour the peace and tranquillity beneath the highvaulted ceiling before returning to the vestibule and the enormous doorway. Now step outside the celestial sanctum and slowly descend the stone steps ... and as you move one foot before the other you find that normal consciousness is returning so that by the time you reach the bottom of the stairway you are once more fully awake and aware of your surroundings in this life.

Terminate session.

Snippet:

The light is more easily seen when all else is dark.

Anxiety/Worry

Now that you are so very relaxed ... your mind is receptive and open to new ideas ... ideas that will help you to stop worrying and enjoy life ... much much more.

Worrying is in fact ... looking into the future ... predicting what might be ... but focusing on only that which could go wrong.

When we care very much about someone ... or something ... it's no surprise when we worry ... It's not pleasant ... but it is natural and it is understandable. However ... if there is no crisis ... or when a crisis is over ... we should stop worrying ... relax ... and enjoy life.

Because everyone needs to relax at times ... even champion athletes who are under a great deal of pressure to perform ... and sometimes need to be perfect to win ... even they need some way to relax and to put things into perspective ... to recognise that it is just a sport and not a war between nations. Because a war is one thing ... and a game is something else entirely ... especially in this atomic age where a war could mean the end of everything. We really cannot afford to make the smallest of mistakes ... and so ... some people are terrified that the fail-safe system will fail ... and that will be the end of it ... all because of some small error ... someone doing something wrong or saying something wrong at the wrong time ... or to the wrong person … in the wrong way. Then everything goes up in flames.

Which is why they have special programmes for the people who are working with these systems ... because what they have to do ... is so dangerous and terribly important that special training and counselling is required. The only place and situation in the world perhaps ... where mistakes cannot be allowed ... and it is comforting to note ... that in almost every other place and situation ... an error is just an opportunity to do things differently later on ... because perfection is seldom needed and rarely required ... and even champion athletes are never perfect all the time ... and sometimes get it wrong. It's like the Navaho Indians who when they weave their beautiful rugs and blankets ... will always leave a knot ... an imperfection so that the Gods will not be angered and think that the weaver is trying to be a God.

But that is another story about what is really important and what is not ... and how it feels to give yourself permission to enjoy the feeling of freedom to feel safe doing those things ... knowing that the world will not end if you leave a knot somewhere ... so that the Gods will know that you are not challenging them ... just doing the best that you can ... letting it go at that.

To overcome your tendency to worry ... follow this simple two step formula.

1. First promise yourself that you will not worry about the small stuff.
2. Realise now ... that it is all small stuff!

We both know that you have an active mind and a reactive body ... and if you think that scary thought for just one brief moment ... then it has been scaring you. We also know that there are other things that you can think ... that are comfortable and calming ... relaxing and reassuring ... thoughts or images that you can use instead ... to help you to relax ... to retain that relaxed calm feeling.

You can let your unconscious mind learn all it needs to know ... to be able to distract you from those scary thoughts … to be able to provide you with those relaxing thoughts and images ... and I think you will enjoy being happily unconcerned ... unable to remember to worry in exactly the same way or at the same time ... so from now on ... when you enter that situation ... you can enter it knowing that you are protected and can tell that part of you that tries to do its job by telling you that there are things to be afraid of here ... that you really don't need it anymore. So it can either go away or find a different game to play ... and remind you instead of all the good things that might happen here or of all the fun things that might occur later ... because those old thoughts and fears just aren't useful anymore.

So you can relax and forget it ... go on about your business ... surprised to discover perhaps that you have been thinking about something else entirely. And you will know at that point ... deep down in every cell of your being ... that you won't ever have to feel that way again ... that it is over and done with ... more rapidly than you expected ... not as soon as you would have liked. You can do it now and you can do it later ... you can frighten yourself with that thought ... or ... you can calmly relax yourself with a different thought. That's right ... so practise and choose ... It is up to you.

Pleasure Returned

Metaphor and suggestion for premature ejaculation.

I wonder if you have ever had that pleasure of looking around a beautiful garden ... and wonder just how you can best appreciate the wonders that are there ... the carefully planted borders ... the colours and the variety of plants all creating a complementary harmony. They bloom each in their own time throughout all the seasons. You can see those who look at everything ... darting from this plant to that shrub so full of wonderment that they really cannot decide which to look at ... which to savour and appreciate first ... There is so much to enjoy ... so much to savour ... the shouts of joyous discovery ... Look at this! ... Look at that! ... Isn't it lovely! ... beautiful ... then rushing on to the next ... so much beauty ... so much colour ... confusing and confounding ... wanting to see it all ... now ... enjoy it all ... now ... miss nothing ... have it all ... so they rush around without taking time to express their real appreciation in a considered and tranquil manner.

There are those who cultivate these delights ... tilling the soil and ensuring that what is offered is of ultimate beauty ... ensuring that the colour and the variety is ever there ... waiting for that time when the garden is open ... the public allowed in ... its pleasures to be enjoyed ... those who take the time ... who make available to us the pleasures that are provided with love and with gentle care ... can watch as those who would enjoy ... take their pleasure ... those who take more time ... relaxing and experiencing as they do each and every petal ... every leaf ... every branch ... so many varieties ... savouring the essence of natural joy in those things which are as nature intended ... they also take the time to seek out the gardener ... the provider of all of this pleasure ... this sensual delight ... and extend to that person who has given so much of himself ... the thanks and appreciation which are also to be enjoyed ... giving and receiving so much more as that interest ... that gentle consideration is rewarded with personal attention and direction to the hidden delights ... the subtle pleasures ... extending the time of pleasure with pleasurable anticipation ... taking the time now to enjoy each step ... each movement ... each new experience ... and learning more of that gardener's pleasure in what is provided there ... pausing to allow time to explore even more than before those areas of pleasure that are hidden from those who rush by ... even trampled and crushed underfoot ... murmurings of pleasure ... appreciation of that beauty and that care ... reverence and respect ... allowing the beauty to embrace and enfold ... that takes them into another quiet and tranquil experience away from the hurry and scurry of those who see only what is there for them ... too excited ... too uncontrolled to share ... and it can be so satisfying knowing that when all is done ... all is appreciated and that appreciation expressed ... that pleasure returned and shared ... that it really is okay to let go in that way ... letting that feeling grow ... allowing those emotions to explode in a surge of delight ... then to tarry a while ... knowing that they really can return again and again ... and each time more is discovered ... the gardener becomes a trusted and beloved companion ... each visit a sharing experience as knowledge grows and each of those pleasures can become something that happens time after time as your subconscious mind finds new and more exciting ... pleasurable ways for you ... with an understanding of those things which are there all the time ... hidden within the realms of your higher mind ... now shown in a wonderful clarity to you as you learn even more about those things that are done for you in that way ... automatically.

So now you can relax even deeper ... in communion with that special and all-knowing part of your perfect mind ... that does know how ... so that the next time you enter that garden ... perhaps to plant the seeds ... that sown with love will blossom and bloom ... I am sure that you too will take the time to prepare the richness of the soil and give appropriate consideration to the miracle that is yours to enjoy ... and I know too that you will remember to recognise that time when the garden is in bloom and the blossoms open ... the soil moist and receptive ... as the bees also know that time ... to allow that conclusion ... that pollination ... that climax to come ... It's completely up to you to enjoy yourself ... or to enjoy yourself giving enjoyment and pleasure ... in return ... as you take your time to pause ... to allow that your love ... your appreciation ... be appreciated too ... and you will ... will you not?

Protecting Others

The importance of belief in self.

Now you will be aware that some people get a lot of pleasure from taking care of others in different ways. Even young children ... who need to be taken care of themselves ... seem to genuinely enjoy doing little things to please those whom they love and care for ... those they want to protect. I am reminded of a friend of mine who when he was just a young boy ... ten years old ... found a baby rabbit that had been hit by a car ... It wasn't badly hurt ... but it was very shocked. He took the little rabbit home and made it a bed in an old box ... with straw and an old jumper ... and he went to the library to get a book on how to care for it. He even spent his pocket money on a tiny feeding bottle. He fed that rabbit every four hours ... setting an alarm clock so that he would wake up in the night. He was so happy as the rabbit grew ... and he gave it so much love and so much attention ... and it would have been so perfect ... if it hadn't then run away ... back to the wild ... as wild rabbits do. He was so upset and he cried when it went but his parents made sure that he knew that it was not his fault ... that he had done everything that there was to do ... and how proud they were of him ... which may explain why he still rescues baby animals and raises them to set them free ... and he seems to feel so much better about himself as a result.

But that's a very different experience from the little girl who was raised by her mother ... a self-styled grand lady who forbade her daughter from ever being better than her ... and made sure that she wasn't. That little girl was raised in luxury and splendour ... pampered and spoiled in so many ways ... but she was never allowed to know that she was prettier ... smarter ... nicer or more talented than her mother had ever been. Somehow ... that little girl knew that she had to do whatever she could to protect her mother from the truth. It wasn't just that it was dangerous in those days to offend the high and mighty lady who was her mother ... the little girl really did want to take care of her ... and make sure that she never felt sad. So ... she acted stupid ... neglected herself and put on lots of weight and whenever she did something well she hastened to explain why it just didn't count ... and that little girl became very good at one thing ... at criticising herself and everything she did. But try as she might ... her talents and abilities ... shone through and she still excelled and accomplished so much in spite of herself ... which made it harder for her not to feel that she had done something wrong ... even years after her mother had died. This was because there was something deep inside her that said that it was bad and it was mean to be better than mother in any way. And she continued to feel that way until one day she really got mad after sitting in a trance for a time ... and realised what her mother had done ... and decided that she had a right to take care of herself as well as she had taken care of others. So she learned how to praise herself as she recognised her own talents and abilities ... her capacity for achieving those worthwhile goals so important to her ... speaking inwardly to herself with that still quiet voice of wisdom that spoke of positivity and self reliance ... reminding herself of her talents and her abilities to love and to care for herself even as she cared for others important to her.

I wonder if you can know how much love she found within ... so much for herself and so much to give and how happy she became about those things that she was able to do.

And when she crawled into her bed all soft and warm ... she was able to allow herself to feel glad about being the person that she was and then to tell her mother she was not sorry that she had grown up to be so content with her life and herself ... that it was now time to be set free and to obey the natural and undeniable yet gentle truth of self-determination using the talents and the abilities which had been given to her that were positive and beneficial ... moving forward now no longer shackled to what was gone ... forever ... growing as the plants and the trees do moving ever on towards the light.

Trance termination.

That Quiet Inner Voice

For use with clients who need to become aware of their own capabilities and gain confidence in their own inner awareness and capacities for self-determination.

As you continue ... drifting ... deeper with each breath that you take ... you can be aware of how little you need to be aware of ... the sounds in the room ... the ticking of the clock perhaps ... the rustle of papers ... sounds outside ... each sound helping you to relax even more deeply ... each word that I utter just a signal for you to become less and less aware of the importance of all that is unimportant here ... the exact meaning of words that are said or not said as I talk to you here ... nothing bothers or concerns you as your conscious mind drifts off to a place which is comfortable and safe ... and your unconscious mind takes on the responsibility for guiding and directing your awareness ... down ... into your innermost self ... aware now of that gentle connection ... communication with that part of you that is the essence of you ... that knows all ... remembers each and every event that has served to shape and mould your unique and special personality ... a part of you that you really do hear as a quiet and calm voice from within ... a voice of wisdom and of truth that is so often lost within the clamour and the clatter of the world ... the demands ... the constraints ... the noise that is those who would have you bend to their will ... Now hear that voice ... still quiet and calm ... but now clear as crystal ... piercing through the fog of indecision and lack of confidence ... unmoved and unaltered in its determination to give to you at all times ... good counsel ... wise answers and solutions to all problems ... for your highest benefit and also those who are special to you ... This is that creative and special part of you ... that wise inner advisor that is always there for you with your benefit and wellbeing always the prime consideration ... a constant etheric part that is you and was you before there was awareness of this existence in this time ... an invaluable friend who must be listened to ... and you will ... will you not?

You can recognise now that value ... that unique capacity and capability that is yours ... has always been yours ... and I really don't want you to know too much about how good you can feel with that intense awareness of confidence in your ability to make changes and decisions in your life for yourself ... no longer allowing others to manipulate you ... to take advantage of you ... You expect of yourself everything that is yours ... that you deserve ... that you are entitled to as a unique and special person ... aware of who you are ... aware of your own talents and special qualities ... always that person who is at the forefront ... always there with a valuable input to every situation ... no longer that person who needs others to make decisions ... you make your own and are comfortable with that ... I wonder if you will notice soon how others come to rely on you to be the person that you are ... confident and self-assured ... an example to those who admire you as you allow those qualities so long hidden ... to burst forth from within ... to astound and confound those who would manipulate and control ... You are your own person ... proud ... confident ... taking responsibility for your own life and wellbeing ... a true friend of your own wise inner advisor ... that is you personified.

The Healing Garden

To be used with clients to enlist their own healing forces.

As you continue now ... drifting deeper and deeper with every gentle breath that you take ... I would like you to imagine yourself in a beautiful garden ... a place of tranquillity and of peace ... Here you are safe and secure ... All around is nature's beauty and colours ... flowers and shrubs ... tall trees that provide cooling shade from the rays of the sun that filter down through the leaves and the branches of these magnificent ancient trees.

A little way off ... just through an archway covered with sweet smelling honeysuckle ... there is a wonderful water feature ... the water sparkling in the sunlight ... cascading over rocks into a large pool below that is filled with water lilies ... Fish swim in this pool ... Now one breaks the surface to feed catching an unwary insect ... And you can find it so easy to relax here ... to let go completely of cares and concerns ... drifting with those thoughts ... that change ... as the world changes.

You continue to relax here ... lying on a carpet of soft green lawn ... the grass cool against your skin ... and you can recognise now that this really is a special place ... a healing place ... a place where so many before you have come to enjoy the peace and harmony ... and the healing powers of the holy men and women ... those who have arrived here through the ages ... sent here by an almighty power to attend to those who have suffered ... and I want you now to just relax ... continue to drift and to dream ... as you wait for your healer to come.

(Allow about one minute to elapse)

That's good ... You really are doing so well ... and I wonder now if you can hear a voice calling to you ... calling your name ... the sound coming nearer ... soothing ... calming ... This is your healer ...

moving close to you now ... a creature of light ... a person of infinite wisdom sent to you from that power that transcends all ... and you feel that power now ... a gentle warming sensation that flows through your body ... spreading from the top of your head as your healer touches you there ... a growing feeling of wellbeing ... moving through every cell ... every muscle ... every fibre of your being ... calming your mind ... and you can feel that healing influence at work now ... stimulating your own natural healing forces within to do their very best for you now ... seeking out those discomforts ... soothing ... relaxing ... encouraging bloodflow ... carrying vital oxygen and nutrients through your whole system ... every organ richly supplied ... your body's defence system moving to seek out all intrusions ... regenerating ... stimulating ... purifying ... healing.

Your healer continues ... moving healing hands over your body ... concentrating on those parts which need that healing attention ... spreading warmth ... that glowing sensation of oneness with the universe ... a growing spreading sensation that cocoons you now enveloping you entirely in its healing light and influence ... You hear comforting words deep within your own inner mind as your own personal and wise inner self absorbs that concentration of positive power ... increasing feelings of self worth ... of confidence ... of your own ability to continue this work ... relaxing in this special way ... allowing your subconscious mind to return you here regularly ... where you can enjoy that healing ... that peace and that tranquillity of spirit ... and you will continue ... will you not?

(Await response and wait for at least one minute or until client begins to stir before terminating session.)

Pain and Discomfort

This script is derived from one I found within a pile of material given to me in 1991 by Michael Carr-Jones. It is ideal for the situation when the client is very ill, perhaps with a terminal illness.

And now ... as you become less aware of your physical body ... you become more aware of your own perfect and pure ... subconscious mind that really does know everything about you ... and that subconscious part of you now opens ... like a blossom opening ... to receive ... to accept and to act on all the positive affirmations ... concepts and images that I will suggest for you ... as you drift deeper now.

As you drift deeper with every word that I speak ... your subconscious mind is fully alert ... active and alive both day and night ... creating new energy ... health and healing abilities allowing your body to rest ... repair and regenerate ... allowing you to adopt all those positive outlooks which are for your highest good and comfort.

Drifting even deeper now you allow your mind to become peaceful ... calm and comfortable ... as your body becomes rested ... at ease ... and now you can imagine yourself in a beautiful place ... a place of comfort ... peace and tranquillity ... of safety and of healing ... a warm woodland glade where you can feel comfortable ... your mind and body rested ... a place where you can return at any time ... and you feel that you belong here ... that you are valued and loved here ... and those feelings comfort you so you are pleased to drift deeper now.

As you drift and move deeper into this place ... the ground soft and springy beneath your step ... the sunlight diffused by the branches and the foliage of the trees ... the subtle sounds of the wonders of nature calming you ... causing you to easily let go and rest so deeply now ... you find yourself by a pool of crystal clear water ... The pool is filled with natural spring water that is heated by nature's own forces ... Steam rises from its gently bubbling surface ... The pool looks so inviting and so comforting ... restful and peaceful and you can begin to see ... sense or imagine yourself easing into the waters of the pool ... You find a convenient rocky ledge that supports you and you feel so light ... weightless here as the soothing waters rise to cover your chest and your shoulders ... You have no concerns or fears ... as the water bubbles around your body massaging and comforting every part of you.

The gentle heat of the waters relax you ... soothe you ... and you sense the gentle stimulation of the swirling waters ... the bubbles massage your skin with a gentle penetrating warmth as the soft sensation surrounds you ... penetrating deep into your muscles ... into your bones … soothing your nerves ...working on every cell and every fibre of your being ... causing you to relax even more deeply than before as the waters swirl and the gentle heat penetrates deep within you ... releasing all discomfort and pain ... washed away by the gentle healing flow.

You relax even deeper now allowing the massaging effect of the healing waters to concentrate on those parts of you ... joints and muscles that have been causing you pain and discomfort ... and you feel those parts relax as the discomfort is soothed away ... you experience a sense of release ... freedom ... peace and comfort that permeates your whole being.

You settle even deeper into relaxation now as the waters continue to massage ... to calm and comfort you ... every part of your body now is free of discomfort and of pain ... you feel so comfortable now as pain and discomfort continue to flow away from you ... your body becomes calmer ... more peaceful ... allowing itself to repair and to heal ... I am going to stop speaking now ... allowing you some quiet time for yourself to continue to bathe in that soothing ... warming water as it massages you and you continue now to allow all pain and discomfort to simply flow away.

(Wait for a few minutes, allowing the client to relax and enjoy the healing forces)

And now ... you are feeling so rested ... comforted ... so completely relaxed ... and you can see ... sense or imagine yourself leaving the warm waters of the pool ... knowing that you can return at any time ... and as you recline now on a grassy bank ... the ground soft beneath you ... supporting you ... you feel warm and comfortable ... tranquil and relaxed ... gazing into the blue of the sky above ... fixing your attention now onto a low cloud overhead.

The cloud acts for you like a cinema screen ... and onto the screen you can see projected the image of your body ... and you see this image with those areas of your body that have been causing you pain and discomfort ... clearly defined ... Now your breathing slows ... as your body rests ... You see those areas clearly defined ... now bathed in a warm and gentle ... soft blue light ... a light that surrounds those areas ... covers those areas of discomfort ... bathing them in a healing aura that begins to shrink ... to diminish ... and you know that as that healing aura diminishes ... that light is absorbing all the causes and reasons for your discomfort ... just as sponge absorbs water ... and you watch as these pools of light grow smaller and smaller ... continuing to shrink with each outward breath ... with each gentle beat of your heart ... growing smaller now ... as that sense of relief ... of release ... increases and you know that you are freeing yourself easily from discomfort now.

Allow the light to absorb more and more discomfort ... drawing it in ... cleansing freeing and leaving pleasurable sensations as the light shrinks down to just small dots ... Now you watch and observe the dots and the pain and discomfort contained within the dots ... and as you watch ... these dots burst open ... changing to a gentle blue mist that flows outward from your body ... rising towards the sun which evaporates them ... eliminating them ... and you feel totally free now.

And as you bring your attention back to the screen ... you see that your body is completely bathed in white light now ... the blue light is all gone and this white light acts as a silky ... creamy ointment that lubricates your joints ... soothes your muscles and cleanses every cell and every fibre of your being ... your nerves are soothed and calmed ... and every part of you continues to relax ... and your perfect subconscious mind is instructed and activated now to make peace ... relief and comfort ... and freedom your natural way of being as it continues to work ... night and day to make this reality ... directing relief as and where needed ... anticipating your body's needs ... doing all that is needed to keep you comfortable and relaxed.

And now ... as you continue to watch that screen ... I want you to allow another image to appear ... an image that represents the healing ... comfort and release that has taken place ... Allow this image to develop ... becoming clearer ... more vivid ... and now imagine this healing image becoming stronger now ... more powerful ... more vivid ... Focus clearly and powerfully on this image and sense ... feel and imagine that it is taking place right in your body in just the right areas ... Let the sensation be one of healing ... know that this is happening right now ... and that healing ... happiness and comfort continue within you whether you are here resting ... sleeping or going about your daily activities ... know that healing ... comfort and pleasant sensations are your reality.

And so it is that healing ... comfort ... happiness and pleasant sensations **are** your reality ... and you realise and understand that your body and mind are always alert ... and if any situation arises within your body that requires your attention ... then that information is communicated to you ... quickly ... accurately and with the minimum of discomfort.

And your pure subconscious mind knows that once attention has been drawn to an area that needs attention ... and that you have acknowledged that pain and discomfort are no longer productive ... it will release them ... allowing you to maintain your feelings of peace ... relaxation and comfort.

I am now going to give you some trigger words ... that will act as a post hypnotic conditioned response ... Whenever you want to boost your positive thinking ... intensify your subconscious activity in producing good feelings ... and wellness ... you simply close your eyes ... breathe deeply ... exhale slowly and say to yourself ... **easy control....** You breathe deeply ... exhale slowly and you say to yourself ... **easy control** and these words act as a conditioned response signal that informs your subconscious that it need to create immediately ... a feeling of wellness ... feelings of freedom ... comfort.

As you leave this place now ... you feel yourself moving into a bright new day ... a brand new day where you enjoy now a feeling of higher attitude ... more positivity ... an almost overwhelming sense of well being ... and you sense calm ... acknowledge that you belong and that you are happy ... that you can create your own reality now ... and the following words ... concepts ... affirmations and images profoundly impress your pure and perfect subconscious mind ... becoming activated now in your every thought and activity ... natural behaviour.

- You are relaxed, calm and happy.
- This is a good day for you ... any discomfort is immediately released.
- Your body relaxes naturally ... each day as you practise your programmed relaxation ... you become more relaxed ... more skilled at relaxing and your deep signal breath and your natural state of relaxation become effective protection against discomfort.
- A new door in your life stands open before you now as you naturally see the best in all situations.
- You deserve to be healthy ... you deserve to be loved and you are a stronger wiser person because of your experiences ... because of the tests and challenges placed upon your mind and body.
- Your thoughts are healing ... nurturing … and you now release the past to make way for a glorious new present moment ... love and healing fill and surround every cell and fibre of your being.
- You are confident and optimistic as you say goodbye to past fears and you embrace change ... accepting that everything is part of your natural evolution ... ultimately leading to your highest good.
- You now release your fears and insecurities and replace them with faith and confidence.
- You are free and you choose to accept peace ... health and happiness … to be your natural condition.
- Your sleep is relaxed and refreshed and you awake to each new day determined to live each moment in perfect happiness and joy.
- You grow stronger and every day at a more subtle level ... you are naturally healing.
- Your cellular memory is focused now on positivity ... on health and on well being.
- Your mind is charged with healing goals that permeate every cell of your body.
- You feel good about yourself ... day and night ... directing healing thoughts and energies throughout your entire being.

And your mind acts now on these suggestions ... concepts and images ... producing a satisfying ... calmer and more productive life as you create joy ... happiness and peace and calm in every waking moment ... learning from the past ... unafraid of the future ... and happy in the only moment that has true meaning for you ... the present one ... a true gift to you.

Trance termination.

Taking Responsibility

Metaphor and suggestion for determining what is important.

As you rest quietly there ... aware now of that gentle connection between your mind and your perfect inner self ... that part of you that has all those capacities ... knowledge and abilities to solve those problems that are causing you pain ... to create for you so many alternatives that are positive and beneficial for your highest good ... I am reminded of a client of mine who came to see me for help with a problem that he had at work.

Now John had a very good job with an insurance company and he had a lot of colleagues working with him whom he regarded as friends ... people he would often socialise with and who came to dinner parties at his home ... He had a very good social life indeed.

John was very good at his job and often he would be able to help others with his knowledge and his enthusiasm. Because he worked with people whom he regarded as friends ... he felt very much that he had a duty to help them in any way that he could. He would sort out his friends' problems because he had a confidence in his own abilities and thought that he could do this so much better than they.

He spent a great deal of his time and energy putting the mistakes and omissions of others to rights ... ensuring in this way that they would not suffer from their lack of ability and enthusiasm and lose for the company valuable business. He defended their mistakes and even covered up for them using his own time and energy to visit clients on their behalf to ensure that contracts were finalised.

His friends did very well by him ... He worked long hours and took on the stress and the pressure in making absolutely sure that he did all he could to help them. After all these people were his friends and true friends will always make sacrifices for those whom they care about.

He failed to take much notice at first ... of the growing and constant headaches ... the tiredness … and of the fact that he had become so short tempered ... snapping at his wife and children for no good reason.

He was not too much concerned that the sexual side of his marriage was now almost non-existent and that his family life seemed to be sliding down a long and slippery slope of constant rows and upsets. His smile had gone ... his energy spent … and he spent longer and longer hours at the office struggling to complete the immense workload that he had almost entirely forgotten was not his but that of others.

I wonder if you can imagine his feelings when one day he was called into his superior's office ... to be told that a review of personal performance figures had shown that he was producing less business and was now below the average of the rest of the people in his department. He was told that because of the decline in his performance ... the promotion that he had been expecting would not be his ... that his performance would be monitored and reviewed on a weekly basis and that he was at risk of losing his position if his performance did not improve.

He went back to his desk ... very upset and confused ... After all ... he knew his job so well and had worked harder and longer than anyone else in the office.

He then discovered that the friend whom he had helped most ... whom he had carried and covered for ... whose mistakes he had rectified ... was the one who had received the promotion that was to be his.

It took a very true and special friend to tell him the truth, and it was with great sadness that he eventually came to the realisation that in taking on the responsibilities for the lives and the problems of those whom he considered his friends ... he had neglected to his own detriment the responsibility that was his ... the responsibility for his own health and happiness and for his own wife and children ... the responsibility to take for himself the time to ensure the quality of life that was his by right. He took a decision to accept the responsibility that was his ... to do that which was beneficial and right for him and for those he loved and cared for.

He had some leave to come and made a decision to take himself and his wife and children away on holiday, and for two glorious weeks devoted all his energies to putting back that which had been lost. As if by magic ... the headaches and the lacklustre feelings just dissolved away as he involved himself once again with the important and valuable things of life. He relaxed as you are now so very relaxed and rediscovered the pleasure of a loving wife and the joys of children ... It did not take long for him to realise the truth and to recognise that he had become obsessed with taking on the responsibilities of others.

He resolved to take care of the most important elements of his life ... his wife and family and himself ... those who loved him and whom he loved and cared for were where his true responsibilities lay.

When he returned after his holiday ... I wonder if you can imagine his feelings to discover that the office was in a state of chaos. His colleagues made it plain to him that they felt that he had let them down ... going away and leaving them so much work to do.

It was with great deliberation that he addressed the whole of the staff that day. He explained to them that he would no longer be prepared to take on their workload and that they would have to accept for themselves the responsibility that was theirs for their own performance. He made plain that he would not interfere in that responsibility ... but that if his advice was required ... he would be pleased to give them the benefit of his experience ... but that decisions taken would have to be their own. He spoke of how they would all need to accept responsibility for their own lives ... no more and no less than he was for his ... that they were all entitled to, as was he, the reward for their own efforts and diligence and they were not entitled to a reward for the effort he had put in on their behalf.

It didn't take long for the office to fall in line with these new rules, and very soon John was back on top where he belonged. He no longer took on the responsibility other than that which was his and his colleagues soon realised that with just a bit more effort ... they too could do well. They learned to accept the advice that John would give ... but also that they needed to ask for that advice and then to accept responsibility for the decision that needed to be made. Perhaps too a lesson was learned that gifts given should be appreciated and treasured and that kindness improves with the giving.

Experience can be a bitter pill to swallow ... the realisation that even friends will happily allow their responsibilities to be shouldered by another while they reap the benefit of labour and effort that is not theirs ... and perhaps you can wonder too that the time given was so greedily taken and then so casually acknowledged.

I know that you will take the time to give to yourself that which you are entitled to ... time to care for you ... not in an egotistical way ... but in a way that will mean that you make those decisions which are right for you and for those whom you love and care for. You accept now without reservation or pause the responsibility that can only be yours and allow others the freedom to choose what is right for them. You wish all around you the same good feelings of freedom and of confidence in your own abilities and capacities that you enjoy ... as you establish yourself as your own person ... that person whom you like and respect ... a confidant of your own wise inner advisor as you allow that wonderful feeling of oneness with yourself to expand and cocoon you now with its calming light of beneficial calm and positivity. Now you are your own person ... are you not?

Tension and Stress

And now we will relax each part of your body a little at a time ... and each time I say the word **relaxed** you will automatically become ten times more **relaxed** than you already were ... each time I say the word **relaxed** you will become ten times more **relaxed** than you already were.

So now concentrate particularly on the feelings in your toes and feet .... just allow all the muscles and fibres in your toes and feet to become very deeply **relaxed** ... perhaps even picturing in your mind's eye what that would look like ... for all those tiny muscles and tissues to relax ... to become loosely and deeply **relaxed** ... allowing yourself to get that kind of feeling you have when you take off a pair of tight shoes that you've had on for a long time ... and you can just let go of all the tension in your toes and feet and feel the relaxation spread. *(Pause)*

And now imagine that this comfort and relaxation is beginning to spread and flow like a gentle river of warmth ... upward ... through your ankles ... and all through your calves. Letting go of all the tension in your calves ... allowing them to deeply and restfully and comfortably be **relaxed**.

And now that comfort is continuing ... flowing upwards ... into your knees ... behind your knees ... through your knees and into your thighs ... letting go of all the tension in your thighs ... as they deeply ... deeply become **relaxed** ... Notice the sense of gentle heaviness in your legs ... as they just sink down limply and comfortably and **relaxed**.

Continue to let that comfort flow upwards and spread at its own pace ... into the middle part of your body ... flowing into your pelvis and abdomen and stomach ... through your hips and into your lower back ... letting that soothing ... deep comfort spread ... inch by inch up through your body from muscle group to muscle group .... The whole of your body becoming deeply **relaxed**.

Now that relaxation ... that river of warmth ... gradually progresses ... flowing upwards into your chest ... into your back ... between your shoulder blades and into your shoulders ... deeply ... deeply ... **relaxed** ... Every muscle along your spine is relaxing ... relaxing all the more ... heavy and **relaxed**. ... Just allow all the tension to loosen and flow away ... as if somehow just the act of breathing is increasing your comfort ... and you become more and more **relaxed**.

And allow now that comfort and relaxation ... to flow into your neck and throat ... perhaps imagining once again what that would look like ... for all the little fibres and muscles in your neck and throat to deeply ... softly ... comfortably relax. ... Let the relaxation sink deep into your neck ... and it gradually flows up your neck into your scalp ... all across your scalp as if it's bathing your head with waves of comfort and relaxation. Deeply ... totally ... **relaxed**. ... And that relaxation can now flow into your head and forehead and like a gentle wave ... across your face ... into your eyes ... your cheeks ... your mouth and jaws ... Just let go of all the tension in your face ... your mouth ... your jaws ... around your eyes ... allowing those tissues and muscles to loosen and become slack and **relaxed** ... totally **relaxed**.

And now allow that comfort to flow back down your neck ... and across your shoulders ... down into your arms ... your hands ... your fingers and your fingertips ... letting go of all the tension and tightness ... letting go of all the stress and strain ... Just allowing your body to rest and become totally ... **relaxed**.

This is your time and a very special time for you .... nobody wanting anything ... nobody needing anything ... nobody expecting anything.

You have now become so deeply **relaxed** ... that your mind has become very sensitive and receptive to what I say ... so that everything that I put into your mind will cause a deep and lasting impression there and nothing will eradicate it ...These suggestions and instructions will always be for your benefit.

Every feeling that I tell you of ... you will experience ... you will experience exactly as I tell you.

Every day your nerves will become stronger and steadier ... your mind calmer and clearer ... more composed ... more placid ... more tranquil ... You will become much less easily worried ... much less easily agitated ... much less easily fearful and apprehensive ... much less easily upset.

You will be able to think more clearly ... concentrate more easily.

Every day ... you will become emotionally much calmer ... much more settled ... much more completely **relaxed** ... less tense ... both mentally and physically.

Every day now you will feel a greater feeling of personal safety and security than you have felt for a long long time.

I want you now to imagine that you are outside a very tall wall with a large wooden door ... there is a large handle to the door ... and as you turn the handle it opens easily before you and you walk into the most beautiful garden that you have ever seen.

This is your very special place ... Take off your shoes and walk barefoot across the grass ... see the flowers ... the wonderful colours ... smell the wonderful aroma of the flowers ... the grass and the trees ... See the browns and greens of the trees ... See the leaves fluttering in the gentle breeze ... the birds singing in the trees ... Now find a place for you to lie down. Rest your head back and look up at that clear blue sky ... where the sun is shining gently and all is well in your world ... and as you look up at the sky so you notice one white fluffy cloud ... This is your cloud … your very special cloud ... and as you look at it peacefully ... lovingly ... so you notice it begins to descend from the sky ... slowly ... gently … floating down towards you until eventually you are enveloped by this wonderful ... soft cloud ... It gently massages your body ... soothing and healing with a very gentle energy and you feel calm ... safe and secure ... You can feel the soothing energy gently massaging the whole of your body ... Now you can feel the energy of the cloud beginning to penetrate your body ... in through the pores ... flowing through your body and pushing out any remaining tensions ... depressions or anxieties ... being pushed out through your fingertips and toes ... All those bad feelings are being pushed out ... all negativity being pushed out ... and you are left feeling calm ... **relaxed** and carefree .... nobody wanting anything ... nobody needing anything from you ... You are calm ... safe and secure because that cloud has placed a protective shield around your body ... protecting you totally from outside pressure ... It is an invisible shield around your body and will remain there.

You can feel your body tingle with pure healthy soothing energy ... You can enjoy the wonderful clear ... pure fresh air.

So take a deep breath and as you breathe out you are relaxing deeper and deeper ... You are relaxing deeper and deeper .... and as you continue to relax feel yourself ... **relaxed** with your feelings ... And should any unwanted pressure come to you ... remember you are surrounded by an invisible shield from the cloud ... that will protect you from pressure ... The shield will protect you from pressure ... the shield from that cloud will protect you always ... Pressure now will just bounce off and away ... no matter where it comes from or who sends it ... It just bounces off and away .... The pressure and stress bounce off and away ... You are protected from tension and anxiety.

You will now go through your days feeling fine ... You will feel the stress bounce off and away ... the more stress outside ... the calmer you feel inside. ... You feel calm inside ..... You are a calm person and you are shielded from stress .... you act in ways that make you feel good ... You now have new calm responses to old situations ... Your new responses will make you feel strong ... calm and free ... You will feel good about yourself because you have new calm responses that are making your days more pleasant ... You are calm ... strong and free from stress ... You are completely free from stress ... You are calm ... and contented and free from stress.

Feel yourself relax ... know that you are in control of your choices ... You have the choice to be stressed ... nervous or easily upset ... You also have the choice to be calm ... **relaxed** and at ease with your environment ... and you **now choose** to experience life in a calm and **relaxed** way and to flow easily with life's ups and downs.

At work or at home the pressure may mount but you remain calm ... at ease and **relaxed** ... You breathe easily and evenly and your stomach is calm ... From now on you will make the choice to relax in any situation ... You will feel yourself breathing easily and evenly ... Now just let this new choice for peace and calm flow through every cell of your body.

You are now feeling very good ... you can feel an inner quietness that wasn't there before. An inner peace ... an inner tranquillity ... and it feels good ... all those tensions ... all those anxieties just lifted from you. ... all you are left with is the peace ... the quietness and the tranquillity and it feels good ... so very very good.

And this peace and quietness that you feel now is going to remain with you and grow stronger and stronger ... This is something you are going to feel very aware of ... You feel the peace now ... and you will feel it getting stronger and stronger as each day goes by ... and the strength of that peace ... is going to give you the strength to cope with anything that happens in life ... You will be able to deal with it well ... because that peace ... that perfect peace that you feel now is going to remain with you and grow stronger and stronger as each day passes.

In a few moments I shall count from one to seven and on the count of seven you will gently awaken and this peace ... this perfect peace ... will remain with you.

Sexual Assault

Now you are doing so well ... allowing yourself to enjoy that feeling of relaxation ... a feeling of being safe and secure here with me. Now as you continue to relax ... breathing slowly and easily ... I want you to allow your own subconscious to show you yourself ... I want you to be watching you ... seeing yourself clearly as if you were watching through a window ... Tell me when you can see yourself in that way ... That's good ... Now as you watch that scene ... through that window ... I want you to know that you are so much in control of that scene that you can make what is happening there go forwards and backwards too ... and also I want you to see that you can easily make the scene brighter and sharper ... or duller and very hazy ... You can make everything fade out completely ... and I want you to utilise these abilities to help you to experience those things that have happened to you that have caused you so much pain ... but in this way ... You can see all of those events happening but remain completely safe ... both physically and emotionally here with me.

I am going to ask you now to watch through that window and see that time that place when you experienced that sexual assault ... and I want you to try to feel all of those emotions and the physical touch ... the smells ... the taste ... be aware of it all and be aware too of the fear that these events generate within ... and I want you to tell me of that fear ... all the thoughts that are going through your mind ... as you watch the whole thing ... watch it fast and then slow it down ... experience it ... speed it up again and go through it at least six times over and over ... and now ... stop! ... stop that scene and allow the scene to be one of the present ... right here ... right now.

Now I want you to hold onto my wrists ... I want you to grip my wrists as tight as you want ... and as you squeeze so hard I want you to see again those images of that person who did this to you ... and I want you to express your anger ... your rage ... your hatred at that person ... Swear and curse ... Say whatever you want to ... Do not hold back at all ... Let your feelings towards him take over ... **louder ... louder still** ... more now even louder ... and now ... you have done so well ... just relax ... relax completely now ... relax.

Now I want you to hold onto my forearm ... but I want you to be gentle now ... gently massage and squeeze my forearm with both your hands ... that's right ... and as you do this I want you to go deep inside and find all the forgiveness that is in you and I want you to forgive that person ... forgive him as you recognise that it is not you that has the problem ... forgive him because he is the one who has the problem ... for by forgiving him in that way you can be free ... free of what he did to you ... Only by forgiving him can you be free ... so say it now ... free yourself of him ... forgive him ... go on say it now.

That's good so very very good ... I am so impressed that you have done that for yourself ... and now you can allow yourself that relaxation ... drifting down now deeper ... deeper ... calm ... **relaxed** ... feeling safe and secure.

As you have faced that scene again and again ... by repeatedly experiencing that scene ... the problems and the pain will decrease ... decrease to the point where they will have no power to hurt you ... You will not be bothered by them ... because each time you revisit that scene ... express your anger ... and then come back to the present and forgive your attacker ... so you grow and experience that strengthening of your inner self ... the regaining of your self confidence ... your feelings of self worth ... Each time you do this you will find it more and more difficult to experience that event ... the emotions and the pain ... The details of that time fade and dim ... and as these things occur so you will become more contented ... more at peace with yourself as you begin once more to take control of your life and your emotions ... growing more positive ... stronger ... with every session when you are here with me ... aware each time of that change ... and aware too that change is not noticeable right away ... but continues to grow as you become more confident ... recognising that you can ... you will forgive him ... that you have no guilt at all ... you have no problem ... growing each day in self respect ... and emotional security ... your unique personality shining through ... returning stronger and stronger ... You are becoming that person you were ... vital ... special ... beautiful ... worthy of the respect ... better than before ... stronger ... more resolute and capable of meeting all the challenges of life.

You regain each day more and more of that personal strength ... that strength becoming even more than before a permanent ... powerful part of your personality.

You recognise now and are fully aware that it was not you who had a problem ... it was that person who had the problem ... This was not yours then and never will be... You have come through ... the same person as before ... but now stronger ... stronger than you ever were.

I wonder now how easily you will recognise the truth of what really happened then ... that you were the victim of circumstance ... in the wrong place at the wrong time ... Your attacker had the problem and what happened was not directed at you ... it was at that problem.

I want you now to watch again ... feel within you a growing inner strength ... a growing self respect and self love ... You are a complete and whole individual ... in control of your life and you see yourself in that way ... in control ... a complete and special individual ... and you recognise too that you have that ability that understanding that will allow you to help others who have been victimised as you have been ... sharing with them your experience ... that of regaining confidence and self respect ... regaining a recognition of true self worth ... a feeling of being special and knowing it to be so very true about you.

Watch through that window now ... and see how different that scene is ... see yourself there growing in inner strength ... confidence ... self-esteem ... and see yourself sharing these positive thoughts and feelings with others ... giving to others what you have held on to ... that which you deserve to have ... that is yours ... feelings that are good ... positive and beneficial ... that allow you to grow and to move forward now with so much valuable new understanding ... Each time you experience that scene through that window ... negativity ... feelings of anger ... rage ... disgust ... just fade and disappear and something wonderful happens ... positive emotions ... self love ... confidence and inner strength just flow back from that scene ... through that window and into you.

What you see on the screen ... is how you really feel about you ... and how you deserve to feel about yourself ... and each time you view that scene ... the trauma ... the negativity and all of those destructive emotions that have held you back ... weaken ... diminish and fade away ... Each time the scene will appear dimmer more difficult to see and to experience in that way if at all.

Soon ... so soon that you will not concern yourself that those changes are occurring ... there will be only positive ... happy ... safe and secure emotions for you ... You have lost nothing at all ... nothing at all ... You have gained so much strength of character ... inner wisdom and a unique ability to understand the feelings ... the concerns of others too ... and that wonderful ability to share ... share hope ... share love and respect for all others ... and that ability that most humane capacity ... to forgive.

Time will show you the immense achievement that will be yours as you look back in time at the window to the past ... to that event ... so short a time when emotions and fear created for you that need to utilise your own special and unique qualities of spirit ... to become what you are now ... then and now ... optimism ... strength ... character ... self worth ... and so contentment and peace of spirit will be what all recognise within you ... part of you ... a person who can and who will continue to grow better and better with each new day.

The Final Goodbye

For use with those clients who have lost someone and did not have the opportunity to say goodbye or say those things that needed to be said.

Contra-indications: Do not use with those who cannot accept the concept of continuance of spiritual being in an afterlife.

Induce hypnosis and use "The Garden" deepener.

In this beautiful and serene place where you are so comfortable and **relaxed**... where peace and harmony are so natural ... you can be aware that it is so easy to relax even deeper now as you listen to the sound of my voice ... each word a signal for you to go deeper and deeper into profound relaxation of mind and body ... and did you know that just as you have eyes that see the world around you ... you also have an eye deep within you that we call the mind's eye ... and just like your physical eyes this eye has an eyelid that can close down ... and as you relax now it will close down shutting out those stray thoughts and images that are not appropriate here ... and it is closing now ... closing ... closing ... and all that is there now is calm tranquillity ... feelings of peace and of capability ... of beneficial possibilities.

And as you relax ever deeper you can be aware that although you are alone in this beautiful place ... many before you have come here to enjoy and benefit from the positive healing vibrations that abound here ... and I would like you to know that you have been so very fortunate to have known that special person who has so quickly been taken from you ... fortunate that you have been able to hold such wonderful memories that have been for you so powerful ... so influential.

In this special place ... you can enjoy today a very rare and special privilege ... for here ... there ... in that garden of peace ... all must pass in spirit as they travel to that place beyond the gate in the wall at the bottom of the garden ... the gate that you can see now through the screen of trees ... overgrown with ivy and honeysuckle ... a gate through which you cannot pass ... yet ... for you have much to do here ... your life to live. You can be aware of the sounds of gentle laughter ... of music and of an aura of peace that you have not yet experienced ... that is coming from beyond the gate ... in that place where all departed spirits dwell between lives ... where even now there are those who have gone before who wait for you ... watching you and lending to you the strength that they can give to you in spirit.

You are now standing before that gate ... Carved and ornate it stands firmly bolted, for you are not ready to enter ... but just for a time you have the gift now of asking those within to pass through that gate into the garden here ... and for a time you can speak with that special person ... ask what you need to ask and know that the answers will be given with truth and wisdom that is no longer constrained and influenced by these matters of this world ... Those beyond the gate have passed through the veil that keeps from the living the truths and the wisdom and they are no longer fettered by earthly constraints ... All you need to do is call the name of that person ... and he will come through that gate to speak with you ... because that person is in spirit and formless ... I don't know how he will make himself known to you ... you may see him as you know that person ... or perhaps you will experience a feeling ... an emotion that lets you know that he is there ... but you will know that that person is there ... in some safe pleasant way and for a time you can speak with him ... say all of those things that you want to say ... ask all that you need to ask ... and know that here there is only love.

It is different this time ... for you know that soon very soon he must return beyond the gate ... there to wait for you ... but this time you can be sure that all that needs to be said can be said and the peace that you seek can be real ... so that you can release him and then continue with the life that you have ... make the choices that you need to make ... positive and beneficial ... moving on as you need to move on in a way which is natural and constructive ... memories now kept like jewels ... beautiful and valuable … that can be taken out from time to time ... that enhance and make special all that is there ... and you will have those jewels that are yours to keep.

Please take some time now ... time to spend with that person who is here with you now ... some private and special moments ... while I wait back here for you ... to let me know when you have completed all that you wish to do there ... and ... having resolved any difficulties ... are ready to let go ... by just saying, " I have finished here."

(Wait until the client responds)

That's good ... Now you need to tell that person how much you love him ... and say goodbye ... feel that love that you will carry with you ... that feeling of peace and calm inner wisdom that is yours from your experience ... Go ahead now ... hug that person ... and say that last goodbye ... now.

And now that person returns through that gate... is gone now ... leaving with you that wonderful feeling of peace within ... calmness of spirit ... a sense of renewed purpose as you now drift upwards slowly reorienting to conscious awareness bringing with you that new feeling of balance ... harmony and peace ... and when you will ... your eyes will open and you can know that what has been done here will strengthen you more each day.

Moving On

Dealing with the loss of a significant person.

It can be hard to understand why someone who is special to us ... has to leave. It can be so distressing to realise that a very special and important part of our life is over and that there is no way back. A chapter has come to an end ... its story told and then ... what is to come?

You were so very lucky to have known *(name)* ... and to have enjoyed such a special person sharing your life and being part of your life and in so many ways identifying with the person that you are.

Now *(name)* ... has moved on ... without warning and without the chance for you to say goodbye and have the opportunity to tell him how much you loved him ... leaving that explanation ... that apology ... and expressions of sincere appreciation that seemed so difficult to say.

As you relax now ... deeper and deeper ... you have an opportunity to recognise and be aware of your inner self ... that part of you that through experience has the capacity and capability to see things as they really are. This is the part of you that asks the question that we all ask ... What is this life? What is its purpose? Why do things happen in this way?

As you become aware more and more of your inner self ... you can be aware too of the spiritual nature of your being. You can be aware that we are all part of a universal plan ... greater than Man ... greater than any one of us ... and whether or not it is clear to you ... the universe is unfolding in the way that is natural and as it should be.

As we face the ups and downs of life as a whole and try to realise that every experience is leading to the fulfilment of that universal plan ... that everyone of us is here to accomplish something ... some particular phase of that plan that is greater than Man ... greater than any one of us ... the universal plan or life force goes on whether we like it or not.

As part of that plan ... you can be aware that you are as good as anyone else and carry the same responsibility for its unfolding. ... It doesn't fall within the limits of understanding ... but is the natural and normal onward march of events that are part of that universal plan ... regarding which we can claim so little responsibility ... and over which we can exert so little control ... You are not responsible for these things which are so far beyond your control ... You can bear no guilt for there is no guilt to be borne ... You have always done your best in all situations to fulfil your part of the plan.

Okay ... so you have made some mistakes ... but you can accept without any reservation at all ... that you were doing the best that you could and no one can expect any more of anyone than that they do the best they can.

You put aside feelings of guilt ... for you are not guilty of anything and you have no need to seek the forgiveness of anyone for what has happened to you .... You know now that there really can be no doubt that you are not guilty of any wrong ... You were then and you are now ... being the best and the most caring person that you can be and take comfort in that inalienable truth.

(Name) is gone now ... but will live on in your special memories of that time spent together ... and you know that you have been so very privileged to know him/her ... and be part of his/her involvement in that universal plan ... Your knowing *(name)* has been a rich experience that has given you so much pleasure ... and that pleasure will be there with you in memory ... so very valuable and powerful ... so different from the experience of loss and of grief ... the feelings of being cheated and betrayed.

Each day there will be for you reminders of *(name)* ... for you and all who love him/her ... and those memories will carry with them the pleasure and the spiritual union that everyone has with that person.

Each day there will be for you reminders of that very special person ... for you and all those who love him/her and those memories will carry with them the pleasure and the spiritual union that we all have with those we love ... to strengthen you as you find peace with yourself in the knowledge that you too have to play out your part in the universal plan ...

I would like to make the point now ... that there is an absolute necessity to live ... not just in the present ... but in the here and now ...

Each day is a new beginning and the world is made new ... Yesterday has gone and we cannot live in the past ... else we cannot move forward ... because living in the past dulls the keen edge of our imagination ...

The past has value in what we learn from it and use in a positive way ... Loss can help us to realise that what we do have is valuable and to be treasured and cherished ... Constantly bemoaning what is lost and gone from our lives ... serves only to hide from us the things that we do have ... and the need to take pleasure from those things.

To grieve for *(name)* is only natural and right ... You will make those gestures that are the demonstration of your sorrow at losing so very valuable a part of your life ... for by those gestures you are moving on ... Pain will fade and the power of loving remembrance ... will become for you and those who love you ... the driving force of your continuing involvement in that universal plan ... that transcends all human understanding .... That understanding lies with the author of the plan and its secret is held from us.

As you relax now ... Deeper and deeper ... feeling safe and secure there in that special place ... nothing bothers you or disturbs you ... as my voice becomes for you the pinpoint of your focus ... and you focus only on my voice ... drifting now ... comfortably heavy and so so calm ... I wonder if you can see that *(name)* ... really can be here with you now ... here just for a short time ... see his face and notice that there is no sorrow here ... and here you can have an opportunity in the privacy of your own perfect subconscious ... to say now all of those things that you really need to say to him ... and to hear said that which you know he wants you to know ... and to do from now forward.

You can say that last goodbye and feel the love that will remain forever with you ... comforting you now and filling you with new purpose and hope ... You know now that your strength is needed by those who are also grieving for *(name)* ... and you resolve now to ensure that the positive realisation of the value of your family love and respect are carried forward and onward.

You can say this last goodbye and with a new hope ... allow him to go now. No longer will you waste what you have ... thinking only of how you feel. You now devote all your energies and commit yourself to taking the best of what is yours and utilise all of your positive energies to ensuring that what really matters ... what is really important … the future is held close.

I am going to be quiet now and leave you for a while so that you can make peace within yourself ... allowing the power of your own inner mind to do its best work for you .... Please let me know when you are satisfied that you have done all that you can comfortably and safely do there as I wait quietly here for you. When you are done ... just say, "I am satisfied".

That's good ... You really have done so well there ... and now it's time for you to leave that place and return to this place bringing with you so much peace and calmness of spirit ... and a wonderful feeling of hope and contentment that the future is there for you to make your own.

Trance termination.

Time on Time

I wonder how Einstein felt when he realised the implications of the concept of his theory of relativity ... of how time and its measure is but an illusion ... its accuracy determined by so many factors that are beyond our control ... It can be like measuring a mile with an elastic rope and then understanding that the cold or the heat can cause expansion or contraction ... and is it not so that a fleeting moment of pleasure can be so short ... and a moment of pain can seem so very very long? ... It really does come down to how and what we feel ... but time moves on ... and that is certain and we cannot go back ... except in our thoughts .... We as humans have a gift ... in that we can choose to allow ourselves the recall of a moment in time ... or to dismiss it and choose another ... or even project those thoughts of experiences past ... forward to a moment yet to come ... the page unwritten ... and then predict what will be writ ..... The finger of fate writes and having writ moves on ... It can be so confusing to find that what was planned ... what was expected was not to be ... and that events occur in their own particular manner ... and in the midst of this confusion when control is not possible ... we can but seek to control by making important ... the mere measure of time within the constraints of our understanding ... to be on time ... perhaps without taking the time to consider why it is important ... and what can be lost and by whom ... and then to whose advantage.

That which can be written has past ... and in the writing is committed to the realms of history ... unalterable ... and yet is it not so that history can be written so differently from particular points of view and experience? ... The experience gained is personal and is coloured with those pigments available ... for if there were no blue ... how could there be blue? ... I know you will know **now** that what is important is ... **now** ... because what was **now** then becomes ... then ... and is no more ... is gone ... time spent and beyond recovery ... Only **now** ... this moment is important and of real value for **now** continues from **now** ... to the new moment of **now** ... because the **now** that is past is **then** ... and then is dead ... I know that you will from **now** ... choose to enjoy each moment ... and cast aside the negative influences of ... Sorry – **then** ... for **now** is special and important ... What is **then** is gone ... what is to come is yet but a myth ... not even a promise ... what is real ... and I **know** that you **know now**.

You **now** are constantly on guard ... and aware of the dangers that can spoil and taint your positive and special moments ... and immediately you recognise that negative thought or emotion that belongs to **then** ... you dismiss and consign it where it belongs and generate for yourself positive and beneficial thoughts ... feelings and emotions that **now** can continue protected with a shield of positivity and belief in yourself ... your special capabilities and capacities to be that person that you really are ... un-hindered and set free from the shackles of **then** ... moving ever forward in happiness and love both given and received ... aware that love ... understanding and compassion withheld is lost and gone and is wasted ... I **know** that you will choose to make **now** special and fill each **now** with love and understanding ... rejecting with ease those elements back then which have caused so much concern ... confusion and unhappiness ... as you recognise too that you can help others **now** ... as you express without fear those emotions that are born of love ... of forgiveness and your capacity to give credit and understanding to those who are special and important to you.

As you do this **now** and **now** again ... your own special qualities and personality will shine forth and so others will warm to you ... feel comfortable in your company ... as they too recognise you have learned a secret ... discover a harmony of spirit within that takes you forward on your journey ... and your byword is simple "**now** is my moment and my life is **now**" ... Changes are occurring **now** ... deep within ... some you will recognise with sudden and pleasurable clarity ... others will grow and become a permanent and beneficial part of your ever growing personality as you become more and more confident ... more and more assertive of your own abilities and capacities ... listening to that inner voice that gives you good and true counsel ... as you cast aside outmoded and inappropriate convention and habit ... comfortable with your own humanity ... personality ... allowing others who are special to you who love and care for you to share too that which they wish to share with you ... and I **know** that you will **know** too that **now** will be special.

You **now** allow people to be themselves and allow them their own priorities ... You no longer get angry because others do not agree with you or meet you own standards .... You recognise **now** that the only value the opinions of others has ... is the value that you give to them ... You no longer get angry because their opinion or standards are different from yours ... as you exercise with ever increasing ease your control over your own emotions ... recognising that reacting with anger is a waste ... It is negative and has no place in your life .... You reject negative thoughts and emotions ... choosing always to be positive ... You are not that person who will react with uncontrolled anger ... Instead of becoming angry ... you now see their point of view and you react with understanding and care .. and are calm ... while you remain assertive of your own convictions and standards ... You react always with positive thoughts and emotions.

And now *(client's name)* I would like you to experience again a particular situation that in the past has seen you react with anger and aggression ... but this time as you experience that event ... I would like you to notice that you are calm ... that you are in control of your thoughts and emotions ... that you feel so much more comfortable with yourself and with the positive emotions that are now an integral part of the manner in which you contend with all elements of your life.

And now *(client's name)* I would like you to really try to get really mad and discover that positive thoughts and emotions continue to calm you and become stronger the harder you try.

Now ... when you are satisfied that these valuable insights and positive messages have become fixed deep in the subconscious of your mind ... there for your own highest good and benefit ... to be recalled whenever you need them ... then you can allow yourself to drift upwards to the surface of wakeful awareness ... You will remember all that is necessary and beneficial for you to remember and open your eyes feeling calm and comfortable as the vitality flows through you now. On the count of five ... you will open your eyes and know that you have made beneficial changes and feel good. **One, two, three, four, five** ... eyes open ... fully awake **now**.

A New Day

A script for use 'ONLY' with those who have been professionally diagnosed as suffering from depression and lack of confidence; an exhortation to take control of thought processes and therefore take control of one's own life.

Induce hypnosis:

As you continue to drift and float all other sounds fade away into the distance. You pay attention only to the sound of my voice.

I want three points about depression to become firmly established in your mind ... These points are what we are going to deal with ... and each point about depression is the absolute truth to you ... Now the first point is that you have a right to be here ... You are as good as anyone ... You are a child of the universe no less than the trees or the stars ... You have a right to be here and whether or not it is clear to you ... the universe is unfolding in the way that is natural and as it should be ... therefore you can accept that there is a universal plan greater than Man ... greater than any one of us ... and so you can be at peace with yourself if you want to be ... and that brings us to the second point.

For that this plan affects everyone in this universe outside of natural disasters ... all depression is subconsciously self-inflicted. That is the second point ... all depression is subconsciously self-inflicted. Now ... each emotion of the mind is reflected in the electro-chemical balance of the brain ... prolonged feelings of depression can cause a chemical imbalance to occur, which usually corrects itself. It can be determined who will usually respond to medication or will respond successfully without it ... in either case, you will be successful in conquering depression. When you do feel well again, you may do so for only a matter of minutes or hours and then the depression may return ... and it may be a little while before again you begin to feel well. There may be four or five such ups and downs before the symptoms are gone for good.

Now the third point has to do with time and the absolute necessity to live ... not just in the present ... but in the moment of here and now ... The third absolute truth has to with the absolute necessity to live each moment of the here and now .... For example ... yesterday ... you were depressed but today is a new day ... Each day is a fresh beginning ... and every morning is a world made new ... a gift to you ... Today is our most important day ... Yesterday has gone. ... We cannot live in the past ... for if we do we cannot move forward ... because living in the past dulls the keen edge of our imagination ... The past ... even yesterday ... can be of value only as a learning experience ... lessons that we can profit from ... Longfellow wrote, "Nor deem the irrevocable past as wholly wasted ... as wholly vain ... if rising on its wrecks at last to something nobler we attain" ... I wonder if you have ever felt circumstances crowding in on you because of failure ... disappointment and depression and said, "if only I could get a break ... an opportunity to start again?" ... Well, remember what Walter Mallone wrote about opportunity, "They do me wrong who say I come no more ... when once I knock and fail to find you in ... for everyday I stand outside of your door and bid you wake and rise to fight again ... Though deep in mire ... ring not your hands and weep ... I lend my aid to those who say ... I can". No shame-faced outcast ever sank so deep ... but yet might rise again and be a man. The sky was overcast ... no stars appeared within the firmament and you were depressed, downcast because the day had brought only frustration ... Today you awaken with the sunlight pouring through your window ... a new day is at hand ... and brim full with new opportunities to build upon the lessons and the foundations of yesterday's failures". Now each of us is here to accomplish something ... some particular phase of the great universal plan that is greater than man ... greater than any one of us ... the universal plan or life force goes on whether we like it or not.

When we face life as a whole and try to realise that every experience is leading towards fulfilment of that plan ... when we take each day and endeavour to make the most of it ... then things do come out alright ... I would say that we have to listen for life to happen ... listen expectantly. Now you have not been listening expectantly ... you really have not been listening at all ... you have been concentrating on your problems and as long as you concentrate on a problem ... then you do have a problem ... because you are what you concentrate your mind upon.

You are what you are greatly concerned with ... now when you let go of that concern ... when you let go of that problem by changing your thinking ... when you say, ... "to hell with that" ... then you begin to see the solution to your problem because your mind is free and you can utilise your capabilities and capacities to make it work effectively for you. Just say from now on, "I let go of my depression ... I develop and maintain a happy disposition every day. Each day I reject the negatives and choose to see only the positive in all things" ... because the only reason that you have stayed depressed is that you have not yet learned to deal with your negative thoughts ... to allow in the positive thoughts of truth, love and hope. Every new day is a challenge, a new opportunity for you to prove yourself in reality ... to be a believer in truth ... hope and love ... that you do not need to feel helpless and hopeless ... that you can separate off and distinguish the vast difference between those events in your life and your reaction to them ... for they are vastly different ... they are not the same at all and you must separate off those events in your life and your reaction to them.

The problem is not whether or not you need a new job ... whether your partner has left ... or that someone else did right ... or did wrong ... or the terrible things that have occurred in your life ... it is not these things at all ... it is your reaction to them ... it is the sentences that you speak to yourself ... within yourself ... such as, "Oh ... my partner has gone ... I cannot go on without him/her" ... or, "I have terrible pain in my back ... I'll never live a normal life again".... That really is the problem for you ... for when you give yourself negative thoughts ... you are bound to feel depressed .. so you have to learn how to turn those sentences completely round, "Okay, so I made a mistake ... but I won't again" ... or, "Okay, so my wife/husband died and I miss her/him ... but I can start a new life" .... Whatever it is that you say to yourself about those past events that make you depressed ... because you have not learned to turn them completely around ... yet! ... When you are in this frame of mind ... you are dead! That is death! ... Remember Lot's wife was told, "Don't look back for you will turn into a pillar of salt" ... but she just had to look back. You are through looking back ... You can only live life to the full during the very moment that you are living it ... and you can enjoy it with the proper thinking. Hasn't there ever been a desire ... an urge to accomplish something you never attained? ... Think about that ... take each day as it comes and enjoy the sunshine

... the laughter of children ... the song of the birds ... the company of friends ..... See all those positive things.

Let each day crowd out yesterday's sorrows completely ... Remember that "He who climbs a ladder must begin with the first rung" ... The Chinese have a saying ... "A journey of a thousand miles begins with a single step" ... As we seek higher and wider wisdom ... each day becomes the next upward rung ... a new opportunity to rise above yesterday's sorrows ... frustrations ... depressions and failures .... to a world made new and given to you .... The oriental poets urge us, "Look well therefore to this day ... Look well to this day".

Now ... in your mind's eye ... I want you to visualise a sign hanging right in front of you ... a sign that has just three words on it ... The words are, "That Was Yesterday" ... That day was yesterday when things didn't go right .... That was yesterday when you failed to turn your negative thoughts around ... That was yesterday when you gave up hope ... That was yesterday when you did not start over as you should have done ... when you were thinking only of yourself instead of the happiness of others and what you could do for them ... That was yesterday when you know that you did the wrong thing. **That was yesterday. ...** That was yesterday when you hated yourself ... but every day is a new beginning and every day is a world made new ... and the past is not wholly wasted ... it is not in vain when rising from the rubble and ashes of disasters and problems past at last, there is something nobler that you can attain ... By replacing negative thoughts with positive thoughts ... every moment is a new opportunity ... and you accept this truth fully and without reservation ... You feel the warmth of truth ... of love and hope coursing through your heart as you relax completely ... confident that there **is** a plan for you ... and that even though you cannot understand ... you must go through those learning experiences that you are going through in order to satisfy that plan .... Whatever experiences you need to go through so that you can allow yourself to be the author of your own fate ... to be in control of your own feelings and emotions ... for this dawn of a new day ... can come only after the darkness of the night .... You cannot have a mountain without valleys ... otherwise everything is a plateau.

The brightness of the sun would mean nothing ... except by comparison with the darkness of the night ... It is only by contrast that we can begin to understand life ... and so ... instead of reacting in an adverse way to those problems and frustrations of yesterday ... you hang that sign high ... the sign that says, **'That was yesterday'** ... You see that sign in your mind's eye ... You lift those problems from your shoulders and you hang them upon that sign and leave them there ... As a result of the faithful practice of self hypnosis and learning to control your thinking in a positive way ... every day becomes a fresh beginning and in the morning the world is made new for you ... a day that truly is yours ... a day without depression ... a day without frustration ... a day without failure ... a day in which you can be more effective in every area of your life than you have ever been before ... **and why? ... because ... you have let go of problems ...** You have stopped letting them control you ... You are controlling your life by turning those negative thoughts around ... because it is not the events of your life that are affecting you ... it is your reaction to them ... You had allowed negative thoughts to create negative reactions to the experiences of your life ... which used to depress you and run you ragged ... ruin every moment of your life.

You have now learned to relax comfortably in the knowledge that you can and you will do your part and continue to do your part.... Is that not so? *(Await response)*

Trance termination.

Confidence and Self-image

When you look in the mirror, what do you see? Is this the real you, or just another visual cue that will prompt your subconscious to deliver a pre-programmed perception of you, a product of past experiences and conditioning?

It is not so much what we see as how we see that commands our feelings of self-worth, and if we have become habituated to seeing ourselves as bad or inadequate then we will perpetuate that perception of self and project it into the world with all the sorry consequences for our quality of life.

The inner image needs to be changed to one that is beneficial and cognisant of all that is good and positive, allowing us to project into the world a person who is confident and aware of his/her own attributes, capabilities and capacities. Expecting that all will go wrong or that people will not like us appears through our demeanour as an invitation for those things to happen. There is much truth in the adage of the laughing child who receives all the attention.

Using the medium of hypnotic trance, we as therapists have an opportunity to implant and then reinforce positive images deep in the subconscious that will play an important part in that process of transderivational search which provides the information to determine that final perception of self which is so important to our ability to successfully interact with the world in a beneficial and positive way.

The suggestions that we as therapists deliver to the subconscious mind of the client need to be positive and constructive, without negativity. Language needs to be precise, allowing no opportunity for the subconscious to reinforce any of the old negative thought processes that have been the cause of the discomfort that has brought the client to the office. Scripted material has the added value of being carefully thought through with particular attention to semantics in order to exclude negative suggestion. It utilises every opportunity to reinforce those elements that will provide the direction for the change required.

Confidence Building

First *(client's name)* ... I would like to extend my congratulations on your decision to seek help and to allow yourself the experience of coming here today .... I appreciate that you made the effort to make an appointment and to arrive on time ... Already now ... you know that you can do that ... It is in fact easy to do ... and what about that feeling of achievement ... how it feels to realise that what was easy first time ... will be even easier in the future ... for it is from positive experience that you learn how to use your confidence in a way that builds and grows stronger every day ... increased self worth ... recognising even more than before that only good and positive thoughts are of value to you ... that negative thoughts harm you ... they actually harm you ... you allow only good and positive thoughts.

It is so very easy to be that person who does not allow for mistakes to be made ... and it can be a comfort to know that an error is simply an opportunity to do it differently next time ... Perfection is almost never needed ... and even champion athletes are never perfect all the time ... and sometimes get it wrong. ... It's interesting to observe that when the Navaho Indians weave their beautiful rugs and blankets ... they always leave a knot ... an imperfection ... so that the gods are never angered and think that they are trying to be gods themselves.

It can be comforting to know that you can give yourself permission to feel safe and enjoy those things that are important ... knowing that the world will not come to an end if you leave a knot ... so that the gods know that you are not challenging them ... just doing the best you can and leaving it at that.

As you go deeper now ... just listening to the sound of my voice ... you can be aware of those comfortable heavy feelings of legs ... of arms ... of your entire body that seems to float in time and space ... those hypnotic sensations that allow you to know that you have travelled from one state of awareness into another state in a calm and confident way ... and I wonder now if you can allow those feelings to continue ... those comfortable **relaxed** sensations of mind and body ... as you drift and dream ... and my voice drifts with you.

You now look to the future in that way that tells you that things will go well ... that you will succeed ... that you are special ... attractive ... intelligent and capable and in this way you programme yourself to succeed and you will succeed. You now look to the future and see only good things and good people happening to you as you move forward to grasp opportunities ... seeing those opportunities ... clearly ... intensely aware that all your worthwhile goals are attainable. You have all the confidence you need to build upon ... all the capabilities and capacities to be that person that you want to be ... special and exciting ... You and you alone have your best interests at heart ... You now take control of your life ... Now ... you are taking control ... You trust your own judgment in all things and you know that you alone have your best interests and those who are close to you ... within your control ... and it is with profound satisfaction now ... that you undertake and commit yourself to your own best interests ... utilising to your highest potential ... **your** capability ... **your** special qualities ... accepting **your** feelings of self-congratulation as you achieve your worthwhile goals.

You find it easy to concentrate on what is important to you ... Your subconscious mind helps you in those ways ... reminding you of your successes ... of your positive abilities ... of all your special qualities ... Others appreciate you more as you demonstrate your confidence ... Your positive approach allows those around you to have confidence in you ... as your confidence grows and manifests itself in your day-to-day success ... Now your creativity discovers new ways of releasing itself ... to become effective and part of your own special personality ... You impress and amaze all with your clarity of thought and expression of new ideas and input to every situation ... once the bystander ... now at the forefront ... establishing yourself as that interesting positive person that you are .... You can now be aware that you are the equal of all ... **relaxed** and comfortable in every situation ... You are realising now with greater clarity each and every day ... that you can unlearn that feeling of fear and lack of confidence. ... You now take a deep breath ... relax yourself from head to toe ... and take the image into your mind of you ... happy and secure ... confident and self assured ... as you tell yourself ... **I can** ... **I will** ...

This comfortable pleasant image soothes your mind, and all fear and self doubt leaves you completely.

You unlearn fear by being positive and realising that the only thing that can hurt you ... is the fear itself ... No longer do you accept fear or negativity ... You banish in their entirety all unwanted inappropriate thoughts and symptoms ... allowing only good thoughts and positive feelings to grow and become part of your special personality ... You do this easily because you are in control ... It will become easier and easier for you to do this as you take control ... and you will take control ... will you not? *(Await response)*

As you go deeper now ... in control ... just listening to the sound of my voice ... your subconscious mind shows you yourself at that time ... that place ... when you really felt confident ... a time when you really felt good ... when you were the centre of attention ... loved and admired ... being congratulated by those around you as you received an award for achievement ... or realised a long standing ambition. It doesn't matter where it was or when it was ... just as long as you felt really good about yourself and about your achievement ... Think of your finest hour ... and get that image into your mind as you were at that time at that place ... You see yourself right now as the centre of attention ... with all others cheering you ... congratulating you ... Now hold that feeling ... allow that feeling to be something that expands .... Now see that special feeling as a pulsating white light ... warm and comfortable ... powerful ... and allow that white light to expand and grow so that it encompasses you ... so that you are completely contained within a brilliant cocoon of pulsating white light ... Feel that warm and comfortable feeling ... confident and admiring thoughts about you and your special qualities and capacities ... Feel it growing ... expanding ... filling your very being with its power and positive influence ... And now ... allow that white light to be absorbed into your body ... as you absorb completely and permanently to your highest benefit all of those good and capable qualities that ensure that from this moment forward ... you are the confident and self assured person that you want to be ... that you are ... right now.

Each and everything you do ... you do better than you have ever done before ... You approach each new task with complete ease of mind knowing that you are ... **relaxed** and in a perfect frame of mind ... calm ... **relaxed** and confident .... Every day your confidence grows ... which means that tomorrow your confidence grows and the day after it grows stronger than before ... and as you practise being more and more confident ... so your confidence grows and becomes stronger as more and more ... your feelings of self-worth become strong and powerful ... Each day ... with each new situation ... whenever you need to ... you take control ... calm your mind ... disregard troubles and you are calm ... **relaxed** ... poised ... competent ... and confident ... You are your own person ... is that not so ?

(Wait for response and then go to trance termination)

Self-assertion

Direct approach for those who have lost sight of the priorities of life and of their own abilities to make choices for themselves.

As you go deeper now ... drifting to wherever your subconscious takes you ... to a place where there is only peace ... calm ... and tranquillity ... and nothing concerns you other than the relaxing sound of my voice ... you can be aware that there really is no reason at all to make an effort to try to hear or to understand each and every word that I might say or not say ... here ... as you rest quietly ... over there ... and it can be a comfort for you to know that your subconscious hears and understands everything that is important to you ... and it's so much easier to just allow those things to occur in their own way ... while your conscious mind can drift to someplace else entirely. As you drift ever deeper with your own thoughts in your own way ... I would like you to pay close attention each time I say the word ... **now** ... This will be a signal for you to go deeper still.

Many people come here to seek help with problems such as you are experiencing ... and they will tell me they have no motivation ... no spark ... no zest ... and my answer to them is always the same ... You have all the motivation that you need and that spark ... that zest for life that once you found so readily available ... is still with you ... but it has become hidden ... lost within a mist of negative thoughts. But congratulate yourself right **now** on the fact that you found the motivation necessary to make the appointment ... and the spark of positivity to arrive here on time ... unlike that person who did not make the appointment ... did not have the motivation to make the effort ... that person is not here **now** ... sitting comfortably there ... that person was unable to distinguish the place from where they are **now** from the place where they would like to be. You have all the motivation ... all the spark and zest for life that you need ... but there is one thing that you don't have ... yet ... and that's self-confidence ... the self-confidence that it takes to set out on any journey or tackle any task ... knowing that you have made all necessary arrangements and preparations ... knowing that you can ... you will complete that journey or that task ... easily ... quickly and without effort. As you go deeper **now** ... just allow your subconscious to show you yourself at your place of work ... see yourself as you start your daily round of tasks ... **now** taking time to organise and prioritise those things that must be done. See yourself calm ... confident as you begin the first of those tasks ... **now** taking the time ... seeing that task through to completion before beginning the next on your list of priorities. If for some unforeseeable reason the task that you have begun cannot be completed you remain positive as you complete that task as far as you are able and then set it aside knowing that you have done all that you can and that you can proceed no further until those elements that are required are available to you. It **now** becomes a new task and you can without hesitation or feelings of inadequacy or guilt continue with the next of your priorities.

Should you be disturbed from the task that you are attending to ... perhaps as a colleague requires your attention to what he or she considers important which needs to be attended to immediately ... you will be aware of a deep inner calmness that comes from deep within your subconscious ... helping your feelings of calm and confidence as you listen attentively and in a calm and confident manner assess **for yourself** the importance that is needed to be placed upon the situation ... and then as those feelings of confidence and calm grow stronger and stronger with every moment ... see yourself **now** asserting yourself as that calm and confident person ... as you make **your decision** ... reach **your conclusion** as to the importance and action required.

You are **now** that comfortable and calm person who is confident with the knowledge that you carry within ... confident in your own ability as you exercise your calm orderly approach to everyday tasks ... and as you do this ... others appreciate you more and their confidence in you grows as you exercise these special qualities of quiet calm and confidence. You will experience more each day the satisfaction and the self pride that go hand in hand with your new and confident manner ... and those things that in the past caused you anxiety and feelings of inadequacy are **now** easy and of no concern. You will be pleasantly surprised at how easy they become ... for you **now** accept that things do not need to be difficult and hard to warrant merit. Each new task and each new challenge is for you **now** a pleasure because you are aware of the simple and inescapable truth ... the truth that you are at your best when you are **relaxed** and that the most that anyone can expect of you is that you do your best. You can **now** be aware also that even champion athletes who strive for perfection ... can make mistakes and sometimes get it wrong ... and even as they do their best ... that perfection ... that great ideal is so seldom required or expected. A mistake is simply an opportunity to do it better next time. You are **now** that person whom you wish the world to see ... aware **now** of your own true value as a unique and special person ... looking outwards from yourself to those around you and aware that you have all that you need to be certain that the decisions you make for yourself are the right decisions for you and for those who are special to you. You **now** take the decision to be responsible and caring for yourself ... for you know that in this way you can be at your best and give of your best for those whom you love and care for and who love and care for you ... and as you do this your true personality will shine through ... Others will warm to you and the bonds will grow stronger as your relationships grow and develop. You are calm confident ... self-assured ... your personality once dimmed within that mist of negativity now shines brightly as those mists dissipate ... and that spark grows bright and clear for all to see ... bright and positive. Experience **now** that good feeling that positive and confident feeling that is yours as you choose to make the right choice for you ... as your subconscious mind does its best work for you without the need for you to know just how it knows what to do.

You now take quality time to be with those whom you love and who love you ... time that means for you that only they are important whilst you are sharing yourself ... and to them you give this time without other considerations. From this time forward your subconscious will remind you as it can ... of those things that are important ... that life is for living ... and that work is part of that life which can also be enjoyed ... but always that you work to live and do not live to work. You now work to enjoy the rewards for your efforts ... and gone forever … is that feeling that tells you that you must feel guilty whenever you find pleasure in life and with your family and friends. You **now** accept fully and without reservation that your subconscious mind will take care of you and all that is important ... and will remind you with a calming constancy of those things that are of lasting and durable value ... that are significant ... and you **now** become a friend of your own inner friend and confidant that you are **now** intensely aware of ... a wise and personal advisor deep within you who has your best interests and well being always at heart. You now hear clearly and unmistakably the voice of that inner advisor ... that long lost friend … and you renew that friendship … a friendship which will now continue always.

From this moment forward ... you are your own person ... you **now** like ... respect and love yourself more ... not in an egotistical way ... but in a way that is beneficial to you as you listen to your own wise inner advisor and trust him/her to be with you whenever needed.

Now I want you to take a deep breath ... and as you expel all the air from your lungs ... go deeper **now** ... and as you turn inwards to contact your own inner self ... you can experience those new feelings of confidence and self-esteem ... that inner trust that allows you to know that you have all you need to be the person you wish to be as those feelings expand and grow to cocoon you **now** within a glow of warming and calming influence that allows you always to be at your best ... positive ... confident ... self-assured ... motivated and full of the spark and zest for life that is there within.

Trance termination.

Self-recognition

As you drift ... so comfortable now ... just concentrating on the sound of my voice ... you can really begin to experience that feeling of knowing that you really can take control ... utilising now your own ability to **relax** ... to let go ... moving inwards now into your own subconscious mind where nothing at all concerns you as you distance yourself from the world about you.

As you continue to **relax** ... all is tranquillity and peace ... recognising now the signs of that deep hypnotic trance ... heaviness of arms ... of legs ... of your entire body that seems to float now in time and space ... free floating now as you drift and leave it behind ... deeper ... deeper.

Now so many people come here to ask me to help them to make something happen in their life ... to make positive changes ... and I tell them this ... as I tell you now ... that those changes are there to be made and that all that is needed here is a recognition of the abilities and capacities that are yours ... to recognise that you really do have the confidence and the determination to do those things.

It is just like setting out on a journey ... knowing that you have prepared well ... everything is packed ... passports and tickets are in a safe place ... all arrangements have been attended to ... knowing that you can and you will complete your journey easily and without effort ... You have all the ability and the capability to do what you want ... to make new and good things happen ... You tell yourself now ... I can ... I will and you feel at ease ... comfortable with yourself.

What has happened in the past has happened ... From these events you have learned so much ... experiences that will help you to know what is right for you ... so you can **relax** and you can let go of all negative feelings and emotions ... turning things around now and seeing the positive in everything. For you ... the glass is always half full as you refuse to accept that you have been guilty of failure ... recognising with clarity that what you did was to do your very best and no-one can ask more that that ... Negative thoughts and emotions have no place at all in your life ... They hold you back ... They prevent you from being that person that you wish to be and that you really can be.

With every day you have learned more through experience ... the best and most effective way of learning that can be ... You are the product of all your experiences ... all of those events that occurred way back then ... You are better for your experiences as you continue to learn more each day about that wonderful ability that you do have to use all learnings in a positive and forward-looking way that tells you inside your own perfect inner mind, ... "I can ... I will".

I want you now to repeat those words ... saying to yourself deep inside where they take immediate and lasting effect ... imbedding now in the deepest part of your subconscious mind ... becoming an integral part of your very being ... Repeat the words three times within yourself ... "I Can ... I Will ... I am the equal of every person ... Each day in every way ... I am getting better and better and better". *(Allow time for client to repeat each affirmation)*

You look back now to those events of childhood and of growing up which have shaped you and made you the person that you are ... You take pride now in yourself as you recognise with ever increasing clarity of thought that you can be selective in those memories that you choose to keep ... to place value upon ... for is it not true that everything has a value ... and for you that is the value that you alone attribute to it ? ... Those things ... those experiences that have no value to you ... you reject now in their entirety ... you cast them away as over and done with.

As you take control of **your life** ... **your emotions** ... things begin to happen the way you want them to happen ... your clarity of thought and your ever increasing maturity ensure that you have all that you need ... an attitude of mind that is positive and forward looking.

As you move forward with your new attitudes ... new confidence in your own ability ... others around you will notice you and recognise that they can draw from you ... that strength that comes from the knowledge that you can be relied on to act in a positive manner that overcomes difficulties ... in a calm and ordered manner ... and you begin to enjoy being valued ... your contribution to all situations ... your opinion sought as you grow and mature into that person that you want to be.

You have all that you need to be successful and you can be more **relaxed** and more comfortable in all situations ... positive thinking can become a habit for you ... for habits are created through repetition ... The more you employ your positive attitudes of mind the stronger that habit can grow ... You practise being positive ... positive and confident ... and the strangest thing happens ... as you act positively and confidently ... then you are seen to be positive ... confident ... It is as easy as that.

Yours is that ability to choose how you wish to see ... with maturity and great pride in knowing that you no longer are that person caught in a trap of negative thinking ... measuring all things in the light of what might go wrong ... Knowing what can go wrong gives you the knowledge which can allow the failsafe systems to be built in ... as engineers do when designing a plane ... or a ship ... or a bridge ... Everything known that can go wrong is evaluated and then eliminated through the application of experience gained ... as you will apply your experience gained ... to your best advantage and highest good.

For you there is no failure ... For you it does not exist as you recognise that the only measure that you need is that of your own success ... Each grain of success is the foundation upon which all success is built ... and this success is now your way ... now and in the future ... as you recognise that fear is just concern that you might lose control ... and that is not true at all ... for to lose control ... first you must have control ... and you choose not to lose the ability that you know is yours to make things happen your way ... "I Can ... I Will" ... these words now become an integral part of you ... part of that internal harmony and peace of spirit that is now yours as you choose to take it and you will take it ... will you not?

Await response and then terminate trance.

Ego Reinforcement

As you relax into this deep and special relaxation ... your subconscious for your protection … takes note of all that is happening around you ... so my suggestions which are all for your benefit ... reach directly to your inner subconscious mind. ... These thoughts and suggestions become deeply imbedded ... firmly fixed in the innermost part of your own perfect mind ... They remain with you ... long after you leave me today ... there to help you begin to make those changes that you wish to make ... for your betterment.

As you relax ... more and more deeply now ... your own self-healing forces are switched on and enhanced ... muscles ... nerves ... the very fibres of your being ... rest ... relax ... Every system slows down ... your breathing becomes more regular ... your heart beats more slowly ... digestion eases down ... so your whole being is at rest ... and now healing forces flow through you ... repairing ... replacing ... re-energising ... soothing your mind and your nerves.

This special relaxation enables you to feel so much fitter and stronger ... more alive in every way ... Your mind is serene and tranquil and you are filled with a deep sense of well being and inner peace ... and as you drift deeper now ... these feelings increase and will stay with you long after we have completed our work here today.

This new-found inner strength enables you to concentrate your mind more keenly ... Your memory improves and you feel more self-assured whatever you are doing ... whatever is going on around you ... so that you have no need to think about yourself ... Your thoughts are directed outwards ... from yourself to the world around you to what you sense about you ... Every day you become more relaxed … more steady ... more settled mentally and physically.

Your talents ... abilities ... all your special qualities begin to grow stronger and more rewarding ... You recognise your own true worth ... and become more aware of your true potential.

This growing inner awareness makes you more aware of others ... their qualities ... abilities and limitations ... You grow more tolerant and your own natural warmth begins to manifest itself ... Friends and relations ... those who are close to you begin to notice this ... They begin to warm to you and your relationships become easier ... closer and much more rewarding.

You feel much more self-confident ... Your will power ... self-esteem ... determination and self-assurance grow with each day ... you feel more comfortable within yourself and within your surroundings ... as day by day these positive feelings develop deep within you ... day by day life becomes more pleasurable ... more fulfilling ... as you feel so much better within yourself and about yourself in every way.

Based on script by William (Bill) Atkinson-Ball.

Self-esteem Boost

Imagine that you are wearing a sign that tells the world, "I am a unique and very special person." You always wear that sign ... that badge and you wear it with pride. Every day you become more and more aware of your assets and the qualities and beauty within you. You now place your complete trust in your own inner mind ... The values and opinions that you accept are your own ... You make up your own mind ... You trust your own judgement ... opinions and values ... relevant ... informed and special ... decisions that you have been putting off, are easier now because you trust yourself and your ability to make the decisions which are the right ones for you and those whom you love ... whom are special to you and rely on you and your special wisdom ... strength ... all those qualities and capacities within you. You admire yourself ... like yourself and trust yourself so much more ... Others too find it easy to like you ... to respect you ... to admire you ... to love you ... but you no longer worry or concern yourself about what others think of you ... it matters only that you like and respect yourself ... You are aware that you cannot please everybody and that the only way to be successful in what you do is to trust your own judgement and to please yourself ... What is right for you will be right for those who are close to you ... and as you do what is right for you ... always trusting your own judgement ... having that belief in yourself ... you now have the confidence to do what you want to do ... Those who would manipulate you and take advantage of your easy going nature ... are now confounded ... aware that with due consideration ... you do what is right for you and those who are important to you. You trust your own judgement and meet your own special and legitimate needs and the needs of those who are close to you and who are special. You meet those needs ... you are independent and self-sufficient ... Changes are happening within you ... changes for the better ... Some you will be aware of now ... Others you will not be aware of until some time in the future ... As you trust yourself more and more ... your subconscious mind will cause these ideas to be made available to you ... ideas for your benefit ... These ideas will be absorbed for your betterment so that you can easily overcome any problem. Know and believe ... that whatever the mind can conceive ... the mind can achieve ... Whatever you believe you can achieve ... you will achieve. ... Every day you are feeling more and more comfortable within yourself and you are becoming your own best friend. Every day you love and respect yourself more ... not in an egotistical way ... but in a way that is positive ... natural and constructive ... and can be only beneficial to you ... Take a moment now to enjoy the feeling of liking yourself and being happy and content with the unique and special person that you are ... Know and believe that each and every small part of your mind ... your body … and your spirit … is an important ... wonderful and beautiful part of nature ... Spirit means your higher self ... that part of you which is inspired ... strong ... kind ... loving and happy ... all of those good and special qualities that are to be admired. Those special qualities are an integral part of your unique personality and are there for you whenever you need them ... If there are things that you have done in the past that you regret ... now is a good time to forgive yourself ... Forgive yourself now and release yourself now from the shackles of those negative elements which prevent you from moving forward. Now you can be that person that you want to be ... If there are things which others have done to you in the past ... now is the time to forgive those others ... Forgive others now and release yourself right now from the past ... You now live for the moment ... this moment ... Now you are that person that you want to be ... a true friend of your own personal and wise inner advisor that is you personified.

Trance termination.

Sports Performance

As you prepare to *(engage in sport/play sport)* allow your imagination to show you a scene ... a familiar place perhaps or one that you can create for yourself ... it does not matter at all ... as long as you can find this place restful and strengthening ... a place where you would choose to be if you felt a bit low or depressed and you wanted to feel better ... If you wish ... you can choose to have somebody there with you ... someone special to you who makes you feel good ... who gives you strength and purpose ... This person may be a brother or a sister ... mother or father ... or someone who is very close to you ... It may be someone whom you admire from afar ... living or otherwise ... By doing this and allowing yourself to experience that place and that person ... you are choosing a place and a person who strengthen and motivate you to your maximum potential.

Some can draw strength from a scene such as a candle flickering ... a water-mill turning ... or a bonfire ... or a mountain stream as it rushes over the rocks. It matters not ... as long as it is a scene which provides for you an inner peace and tranquillity and gives to you a special feeling of confidence and inner strength of purpose.

So now *(client's name)* imagine yourself at that place... at peace with your own inner self ... any maybe with that special person ... and allow that special feeling of calm and confidence ... of tranquillity of spirit to grow and to expand ... as you experience it ... breathe in the essence of it ... breathe in the clear air ... absorb the powerful and positive vibrations and with each breath ... you can feel that strength and purpose ... feel your mental and physical being strengthening ... experiencing now that surge of energy pulsing through your body as your powers centralise ... as your mind focuses intently on the task at hand ... your concentration and your energies vibrating and pulsing with positive intent and purpose ... your mind and body in perfect tune as you prepare for that moment when all your energies both physical and mental will be in harmony and unison ... as your mind sees you completing the *(race/task/performance)* ... achieving your goal ... a winner ... a champion. As you do this feel yourself gaining in strength and health ... increasing your vitality ... taking all that you need physically and mentally from this experience ... feeling better and stronger ... more alive ... more confident in your ability to achieve ... to win ... to overcome.

Practise this for just a few minutes each and every day ... actually drawing the strength and the vitality ... both physically and mentally from whatever helps you ... Know that you can do all that you need to do ... whatever you want to do ... whatever you believe you can do ... You can do it ... if you allow your mind to accept that you can do it ... You can do anything that you want to do if you want it enough and you believe in your own abilities and capacities for greatness and for achievement ... Practise this and then practise some more ... for a few minutes each and every day ... you practise to train your mind to give you the best opportunity and the positive belief in your ability to prevail ... Once you have done that ... you can relax ... confident and assured in the knowledge that you have prepared yourself in the most effective and diligent way possible to be the best that you can be ... the best that you can ask yourself to be. Know and believe that ... if it is attainable ... if it is realistic ... then it is achievable ... that what your mind can conceive ... it can achieve. Whatever you believe you can achieve. Work on believing it ... and as you believe it so will it be ... and you will achieve it.

When you are in competition ... before you make a single move ... you can visualise in your mind a successful outcome ... visualise what you wish to happen ... happening for you ... what you need to do to do well ... for you to succeed.

Practise doing this every day as part of your training and preparation ... and never make a move when you are actually competing without visualising a successful outcome ... Concentrate on what will happen next ... on the next few minutes or the next few seconds ... What happened before does not concern you at all ... It is of no value to you as you shut out from your mind all that is not important to you in your quest for excellence ... Visualise with all your strength and concentrate on only that which is important ... the present moment and the immediate future ... on what will happen next ... Shut out all that is unimportant and irrelevant ...

concentrating on that special moment as all of your abilities and strengths ... concentrate and unite in perfect harmony ... providing for you the perfect balance of concentration ... of positive tension and calmness and clarity of thought ... your body and mind perfectly attuned to provide you with maximum and most effective concentration of effort both physically and mentally ... Concentrate on that future and concentrate on making it happen ... You have all the resources you need to perform at your very best and you know that you will perform to your highest potential ... You have excellent powers of judgement ... Your decision-making will be at its optimum... You will be clear and definite ... and in excellent form both mentally and physically ... you will have all the determination ... confidence and stamina to perform at your best and for as long as you need in order to achieve your highest potential ... You believe in yourself ... believe in your ability ... Whatever you do you will do well and you will do it better than you have ever done it before ... You now believe yourself to be a winner. You **are** a winner.

Trance termination.

Steel Ball

While you are resting in this very pleasant way ... I want you to imagine something ... I want you to imagine that you're looking at a steel ball ... resting at the top of a gentle slope ... Just imagine that now ... You're looking at a steel ball ... resting at the top of a gentle slope ... and as you look at it ... so the ball begins to roll slowly down that slope ... It moves slowly ... and follows a very straight course as it moves ...

But now I want you to imagine that a little way ahead of that steel ball ... and off to one side of the track ... you can see a strong magnet ... and as the ball is rolling towards the magnet ... so it enters into the magnetic field ... and the magnet pulls on the steel ball ... not enough to make it stick to it ... but enough to make it change its course ... The steel ball is now rolling in a completely different direction from its original path.

Now there's a reason for imagining this ... because your pathway through life is like the path taken by that steel ball ... In the beginning your pathway through life was set ... You were following a course that was right for you ... It was comfortable ... It was right for you ... It **felt** right ... but you soon found that you were being influenced by other people ... acting like magnets ... trying to pull you off course ... trying to make you change direction ... In short ... they made you feel that your way was wrong ... They wanted you to conform to **their** ways ... and follow **their** course of action ...

By trying to please them ... you changed your course ... and have been following a way that is not what you originally set for yourself ... The result has been that you have felt uncomfortable ... It has **not** felt right ... and you have consequently felt that you have lost your individuality through trying to please other people ... And this has been the problem ...

So let's see what can be done about it ... Let's return to our picture of the steel ball and make a few changes ... Once again ... imagine that steel ball at the top of the slope ... but this time as you look at it ... see it grow to double its size ... and weighing twice as much ... Now see it rolling and see what happens ...

It approaches the magnet ... and the magnet tries to pull on it ... but this time ... the ball is too heavy ... and too big ... and does **not** deviate from its course ... It keeps on rolling in the same direction ... The influence of the magnet has not been strong enough to affect the ball ... It just rolls straight past ... These simple changes were enough to overcome the problem.

For you to overcome the problem it is not necessary to grow in size ... or put on weight ... but you can grow in strength ... and in power ... and you can do this easily ...

As you rest there now ... I want you to realise something ... and realise it well ... understand it ... and acknowledge it ... It is not your purpose in life to become a carbon copy of someone else ... You are an individual in your own right ... You have your **own** opinions ... You have your **own** personality ... These things are right for **you** ... No other person has the right to try to take these things away from you ... to make you conform to their ways ... You are a person in your own right ... a complete person ... and they must either accept this fact ... or go on their way ...

Your individuality is precious ... It must be protected ... and you can protect this with your own strength ... Your strength has been weakened by the influences of other people ... but that strength is still there ... It is within you now ... so now is the time to rediscover it ... and let it grow ...

So as you rest there now ... just imagine yourself as being strong ... strong enough to withstand the influences of other people ... strong enough to stand on your own feet ... Imagine you are that strong now ... and as you imagine it ... **feel** that strength ... It's there ... You can feel it ... Feel the confidence that goes along with it ... Feel yourself able to speak out ... able to defend your own individuality ... Feel these things now ... because as you can now feel them ... you know they are there ... You already have that strength ... It's there ... You can feel it ... so you know it's there ... Acknowledge it ... Welcome it ... It's yours ...

Now that you have experienced these things ... you can recognise them and use them ... Now that you know they are there ... you can become more aware of them ... Because of this ... you already feel stronger and more able in yourself ... And this feeling is going to remain with you ... and become stronger as each day goes by ... No longer are you influenced into a wrong course by other people ... No longer do you allow your individuality to be taken away from you ... It is precious ... It is yours ...

In a few moments now ... I am going to count up to seven ... and on that count of seven ... you will awaken feeling calm happy and **relaxed** ... You will feel stronger in yourself ... and determined ... very determined to protect your own individuality ... So on the count of seven awaken ... feeling calm ... happy and very **relaxed**.

One ... **two** ... **three** ... **four** ... **five** ... **six** ... **seven**.

Attributed to:

Hugh & Sally Ann North

I Would if I Could

Now as you begin to listen to my voice I would like you to close your eyes ... relax ... let go and let my voice make all the effort necessary ... and as you relax for the next few minutes you let it become a pleasure .... Begin **now** to enjoy the feeling of being able to choose to relax ... to let go ... and to be able to go inside and turn the world off.

As you relax for the next few minutes you are going to learn to enjoy ... gradually ... effortlessly ... and settle into a state of hypnotic sleep ... It is an ability your mind already has inside to settle into a deep relaxed state.

When you came in today ... you had a dream in mind ... something you wanted to make happen in your life ... "I would if I could" has an ending now ... The words that go through your mind ... many times a day ... comfortably ... are ... "I can" ... You believe it ... you begin to feel the pride ... the confidence that makes it all happen.

You begin to feel comfortable with your past ... and your past provides many valuable experiences for you ... many learnings for you ... so as you relax and let your body go ... you refuse to build your life on any form of guilt ... It has no value to you .... What you did in the past was the best you could do at the time. The very best effort you were able to make ... The only reason you know that is because you are better now ... You are better now because you see yesterday through today's eyes. You have matured and grown. ... You understand that there is no value in guilt ... only learnings and experiences have value for you.

Your childhood programming and experiences were controlled by circumstantial accidents ... so keep the pieces you like and agree with ... but any feelings ... any doubts or fears that might live inside you ... anything you don't like about your feelings and attitudes ... those things are not yours ... they happened to you by accident ... you do not need them ... You reject them as over and done and gone.

Now each day happens ... your way ... You mature into that attitude easily ... and new experiences help you to mature into the kind of person that you want to be ... and you honestly believe that you have all the resources you need to succeed ... that you can have all the things you need to complement your success ... You feel this now and increasingly every day.

For now ... relax and experience that attitude ... for what you are doing right now is choosing to turn the world off ... to go inside ... to relax ... to feel a sense of control greater than you have ever had ... That is a reality ... Keep it ... Use it.

You are going to begin to believe that positive ... successful experiences from the past contain valuable emotional strength and depth that you have earned ... Those feelings ... those emotions belong to you ... and just like a familiar song ... or photograph ... positive emotions will bring back buried emotion, ... bring back feelings you think you have forgotten about ... spontaneously ... They will come back by accident throughout your day ... Realise that positive memory pictures can flash into your mind and carry with them the same pride ... the same happiness you felt at the time of the original experience months or years ago.

Those feelings belong to you ... so begin to enjoy feeling the best memories as they begin to occur to you ... For now relax ... let your body go ... feel your body relaxing easily ... a melting sensation flooding your body ... Relax deeper and deeper as you listen to me and let the world fade away ... and as you listen to me ... some of those positive images will flow through your mind ... You are going to use the best within you ... If you ever felt pride ... confidence ... courage ... success and a need to be something special you still own those feelings and attitudes ... You let them come forward as an honest active part of your life ... on purpose. Use your feelings or you lose them ... They are so valuable ... You choose not to let them go.

I want you to begin to practise seeing things as they really are ... You are maturing and you will find great pride in doing that ... You begin to realise that the final choice ... as to how you are going to feel in any situation ... is always yours ... No one can make it for you ... No one does anything to you ... It is your choice as to whether you are going to allow them to control your life in any way ... shape or form. It is your choice ... not theirs ... You are unique as a person ... You are one of a kind ... You will find that people may do what you do but no one can do anything ... no one can ever do it the way you do things ... You are and have been very special from birth and there is no reason in the world to doubt your individual value at any point in your life ... Enjoy that feeling ... It is real.

Failure does not exist ... There is no such thing ... Only your degree of success ever needs to be measured by you ... and even your smallest degree of success is a seed for the future ... It will grow with any attention at all that you give it ... Fear is always a fantasy ... success is always real and is tangible.

You alone are going to decide which choice to make ... Relax now ... Remember, "I would if I could." "I would" ... is a dream and a very good dream. "If I could" ... is the search for a plan or a way to make it happen for yourself ... "I can" ... is the harmony of all the feelings and thoughts that make your life happen ... on purpose ... successfully.

When you hear my voice ... relax ... Let it feel good ... Believe it ... Don't waste my time or yours ... Make it happen ... Make your life happen on purpose ... Each and every suggestion you have heard me utter will register deep within your subconscious mind.

On the count of five ... your eyes will open sparkling clear ... your mind feeling alert.

One ... **two** ... **three** ... **four** ... **five**.

Trance termination.

Love, Truth and Understanding

An intervention for those who have lost trust.

As you drift deeper now ... paying close attention only to the sound of my voice ... you can be aware of how comfortable and heavy you feel as you relax so completely ... As you continue to relax you can also be aware of how easy it is for you to communicate with that innermost part of you ... that is the very essence and substance of the person that you really are ... Here you can address all your hopes and ambitions and know of your strengths and capabilities.

You have been aware now for some time of your own inner advisor and have begun to listen more closely than before to that voice within that really does give you good counsel ... that part of you that knows all about you and recognises too those factors that make you the person that you are.

This is the part of you that can make all of those changes that you wish to make in the way you have been thinking and the manner in which you resolve all situations ... Changes for the better have been occurring within as they are occurring now ... Some you are already aware of ... Others will be recognised as you find new and more positive ways to deal with all situations and all people.

You no longer accept the negative view ... To you the glass is always half full ... Negative thoughts and emotions are damaging to you and in accepting a negative you always hurt you ... Yes ... you actually hurt yourself ... Whenever you experience a negative thought or emotion ... your subconscious mind is ready and will help you to instantly turn that thought around to one that is beneficial and serves your best interests.

Lessons are learned from mistakes ... A mistake is simply an opportunity to get it right next time ... and you know that you would never repeat a mistake with full conscious knowledge .... Mistakes are repeated at a subconscious level in the manner of habit ... but from this moment forward you will be totally aware of each and every lesson that you have learned and if you repeat a mistake that has hurt you and those whom you love ... then you will be doing it deliberately ... and that is not the same at all.

You have always done the best that you can as the person that you were and because that is the way your life's experiences have influenced you ... and so you have no need to feel guilt or shame ... You now forgive yourself for those past mistakes and use the positive value of those lesson so painfully learned to carry you forward as that person who has recognised the importance of trust ... fidelity and truth ... and the value of acceptance of who you are and those things that are yours.

Whenever you experience feelings of wanting those things that you really do not need or that you perceive to be better than what you do have ... your inner advisor will ensure that you hear the truth in no uncertain terms ... You will be reminded of what you do have ... and you will find comfort and contentment in the knowledge that you are loved and respected ...

In this way ... you will enjoy life and its joys so much more ... You will be **relaxed** and comfortable with yourself knowing that you really do not have anything to prove ... You will be confident in your own capabilities and capacities ... and others too will be aware of your calm and confident attitude towards life in general as your true warmth and personality shine through ... You will find that others seek you out for comfort and reassurance ... You refrain from giving advice however ... for you are aware that advice given usually begins with "If I were you" ... You understand that unless you can stand in another's shoes ... then you cannot see things from where they are and you counsel them as you counsel yourself to listen to their own inner voice that will tell them too which is the right way ... accepting the responsibility for their life as you accept those responsibilities that are yours ....

You cannot be privy to the thoughts of others ... and you understand that a silence can never be recognised as either a confirmation or a denial of what you think ... and you choose always to recognise the positive and beneficial interpretation that your subconscious mind will provide you with ... as you recognise too that your subconscious can and will provide you with natural and appropriate caution.

As you leave here today ... you go forth into the world looking forward with a new and determined optimism ... for you are armed now with new knowledge and understanding of that person that you are ... unique and special ... your real self ... confident in your own abilities to be true to those values that really are important and to recognise what is false and inappropriate ... You can give love ... for now you love and respect yourself for the person that you are and you will be happy with all that you do have ...

Yesterday has gone ... and with it is gone all the influences that could make it different. Tomorrow is but a myth ... that we can colour with imagination ... but today ... this very moment ... all is real and for this moment we live ... and then ... that too is gone ... either seized upon and enjoyed ... or wasted. You can choose too which reality is yours ... and you will ... will you not?

(Wait for response)

Each new day is a gift ... every morning a new beginning ... We are promised only the moment of our existence and that wonderful moment ... **now** ... is all that we have and all that we need.

Trance termination.

Smoking Cessation
Single Session Stop Smoking Therapy Method

Table of Contents

The Smoking Gun

Here in Britain the use of hypnosis in stop smoking therapy has been acknowledged by the British Medical Association as the most effective help available to those who are addicted to smoking.

When I first began in practice ten years ago, I, in my inexperienced way, followed the format that others had passed on to me, using the form of 'magic words' that were the scripts that had been given to me.

Those who came to me for help were all treated with the same format: hypnosis was induced and the scripted material delivered, with some success. But there were the failures. I remember one eminent practitioner propounding the view, "It's not you the therapist who fails, but the person who came to you with the purpose of quitting smoking."

For some time I went along with that view for, inasmuch as we all must take responsibility for our own lives, it is the smoker who has the ultimate responsibility for their own health and if they choose to endanger their life, it is only too easy to say when they become the victim of their folly, "It is your own fault. You knew that smoking was dangerous."

If that is true, and of course it is, it can also be a get-out for the therapist who does not apply his mind and his training to determining the best form of help possible for the client. The client of course will be aware that he is the one who will or will not be successful. He will also be aware that he came for help because he needed it. It would therefore be remiss of any therapist not to offer the most effective help available.

So what form should our help take? Everyone is different: their needs and their aspirations are unique, and if that is accepted, then it is apparent that therapy must be entered into with the uniqueness of each client firmly in mind. Michael Yapko says, "*Use of scripts robs hypnosis of its real potency, the strength derived from the recognition and use of each individual's unique experience.*"

The idea that a strictly regimented therapy session applied with vigour can be successful in all cases has to be seen as a nonsense and often doomed to failure. We as therapists must have some sort of structure that we can work within, but that structure must be pliant and adaptable. *Scripts, therefore, should be adaptable. They are not in themselves a magic formula which incanted in hypnotic trance style will instantly turn lead into gold. Utilise the special fears and motivations of your clients and build these into the script as appropriate.*

Over the years, my methods have obviously been evolving and now I believe that I have reached a point where my strategy is effective within my capabilities and that my responsibilities are largely satisfied. I do my best to help that person who is placing so much trust in me, because what I do or do not do will have a significant effect on the quality and the duration of that person's life.

For years, perhaps, the client has been destroying the integrity of his very being. As Yapko says, "*Clearly a smoker is in a physically dissociated state. How else could one be oblivious to the physical damage associated with breathing toxic fumes.*"

Smoking kills, it maims and it destroys quality of life not only for those unfortunates who have unwittingly become entangled in this web of addiction, but also for those who are the family, friends and dependants of that person.

If you, the therapist, can help your client to live longer and enjoy improved health and vitality, then you will have also provided a huge and invaluable service to the client's family and friends. If you can help a child to have mum or dad around for as long as is naturally possible instead of losing that person to an early smoking-related death, then that knowledge can give you joy, satisfaction and justifiable pride.

I have a particular grudge against the tobacco companies who, without conscience, continue their appalling business in pursuit of profit. I hold them largely responsible for the death of my father who was encouraged at an early age to believe that smoking was not harmful, but was in fact beneficial. He was just 55 years old when he died, and I stood by his hospital bed as he struggled for each and every breath until his strength just gave out. I am one amongst millions who can justifiably feel angry that the tobacco companies have been allowed to continue their business to this day.

In the following pages I aim to give an insight into what I consider the most effective strategy to help smokers kick the habit and enjoy their full quota of years filled with good health. I invite you as a therapist to use the fruits of my experience and apply my methods to help your clients. But I would also encourage you to continue, as I have done, to add to what is already there, in the ongoing quest to achieve the best results for those who seek our help.

It is not my intention that this work should allow a complete novice to set himself up as a specialist in smoking cessation. It is necessary that a full understanding of the influential forces that are at work be understood in order that these "tools" be most effectively used for the benefit of those who seek help.

If you as a therapist, having read my book, become more effective in helping your clients, then my motive for this undertaking will have been achieved. Should all of us continue the process of refining the tools that we have available to us, then our ability to help those who wish to make changes will constantly improve. Knowledge is just a stepping stone to greater understanding, so further developments are both essential and exciting.

I trust that all smokers who read this book will be persuaded of the danger that they are placing themselves in by continuing to smoke and will as a result choose to take responsibility for their own health and life, thus depriving the tobacco industry of more victims.

Client Education

A good place to start is at the beginning, and in this situation this relates to the very first cigarette that your client smoked. Ask him to think back to that first cigarette and tell you exactly how it all happened. Usually peer pressure is the overriding reason why it began. (*Whatever the answers, they will invariably point to the association with being grown up, one of the crowd, being more sophisticated and mature, establishing independence.(Allen 1997)*

Often we are in a hurry to achieve adulthood when we are in our early teens. So many changes happen to us during this period when the hormones in our bodies are running riot. Pubic hair begins to sprout, breasts begin to fill out, and the first interest and clumsy encounters with the opposite sex occur. We begin to project ourselves in the way that we would like to be seen, as adults, and can no longer tolerate being thought of as a child, but at the same time lacking the confidence or experience to be a complete adult. So we look for ways to affirm our desired status; means of demonstrating that we really can be adults. It is accepted that adults smoke. With our rational consideration reject any suggestion that we are anything but that which we aspire to become. Trying to talk sense to a teenager can be a frustrating experience, as any parent will confirm!

The beginnings of addiction

Tobacco companies are well aware of the addictive nature of tobacco and thus target their advertising accordingly to young people, promoting cigarettes to be socially acceptable as a indication of sophistication and maturity.

Heroic figures are portrayed enjoying the pleasure of riches and fame, striding through every situation with that air of confidence and success that attracts the beautiful woman or the handsome man.

At this age fantasy is so easily mistaken for reality and we are so gullible and naïve.

It is so easy to believe as teenagers that we are invincible, and the suggestion that we might become addicted and dependent on cigarettes seems ridiculous. This is the age when we really do know it all, but this is an illusion. The harsh reality is that we are too young to be wise and too old to be told. Parents everywhere will know exactly what I mean as they experience the frustration of watching their sons and daughters making the same old mistakes as they did. And did their parents also try in vain to pass on the lessons that they had learned through experience? In the rush to take on the mantle of adulthood, so many youngsters walk straight into the trap set by the tobacco industry.

Drag and cough

When that first cigarette is remembered, I have yet to meet anyone who, hand on heart, can state that the experience was a pleasant one. As the harsh cigarette smoke is taken into the lungs, the effects are predictable. Dizziness, nausea, coughing and spluttering all accompanied by a foul taste, are what most admit to experiencing, but, determined to be seen as one of the gang and not wishing to become isolated from their peers, these young people strive to endure what is perceived as some sort of initiation into approaching adulthood.

The survival instinct

The reaction of dizziness, nausea etc., to the cigarette smoke is one that is generated by the subconscious mind as it strives to carry out its prime function, that of 'survival'. It is in effect sending a clear message as it deploys its defences against the poison that has been introduced into the body. "Stop now. You are poisoning yourself", it shouts as it promotes the vomit and cough response in its efforts to expel the substance which it recognises as dangerous.

Dizziness and disorientation are experienced as the brain is suddenly deprived of its oxygen supply. The delicate taste buds in the mouth react violently in protest at the foul mixture which leaves that unpleasant taste which lingers long after the event. The heartbeat quickens adding to the anxiety that is part of that warning system that alerts us to imminent danger.

The human body is a wonderful miracle of engineering. Each and every part of its function is controlled and regulated by the subconscious without any conscious consideration at all. Our heart pumps oxygenated blood around our body. The liver, kidneys, the brain, every cell, each molecule is monitored and regulated precisely and without pause. The chemical balance of the organism is precise and specific and it is part of the function of the subconscious to ensure that the correct chemical constitution is maintained.

When that first cigarette smoke is introduced the chemical balance is placed in jeopardy, and so those defence mechanisms are activated to protect the integrity of that delicate balance, but the young person is so determined to be one of the gang that he continues the assault on his own defences so that the subconscious programming becomes corrupted and begins to accept the new chemicals being introduced as necessary for its survival.

Now in order to ensure that this newly accustomed nicotine level is maintained, it sends out a signal, a demand for new supplies when the level drops, in the same way as it sends out a signal that we recognise when we experience hunger or thirst or feel too hot or too cold. These signals are designed to prompt us to eat or to drink, take appropriate action to get warm or to cool down. By their very nature they create discomfort which motivates us to take action to remedy that unpleasant sensation. The more nicotine the system becomes accustomed to, the more demands will be signalled. This is what we recognise as nicotine craving and addiction.

The subconscious has become fooled into a belief that it must ensure that the nicotine supply is maintained and a new 'part' of a person's survival programming is created, its sole purpose to do everything necessary to ensure that supply. To keep the smoker smoking; to maintain an addiction to nicotine. *For many people, a pack of cigarettes was the only friend they had. (Citrenbaum, King & Cohen 1985)*

Chemical content

There are over two thousand chemical compounds in tobacco smoke. Around thirty of those chemicals are known carcinogens and many are lethal poisons. We are all aware of the most common chemicals, nicotine and tar, but what of the others?

Arsenic is present in tobacco smoke, as is also cyanide, ammonia, benzo-pyrene, carbon monoxide and prussic acid. Added to this are the insecticides and chemical fertilisers sprayed on the tobacco crops. All these chemicals and many more are present in cigarettes and other tobacco products and now are absorbed into and pollute the tissues of the smoker's body.

Arsenic and cyanide! Both of these substances are instantly recognisable as extremely poisonous to humans. Are you aware that nicotine is one of the most poisonous substances known to man? Why, if you were to extract the nicotine from one cigarette and, with a hypodermic, inject it directly into a vein, you would be dead in seconds! There is enough in that one cigarette to kill a horse!

"It helps me to relax"

Nicotine is a recognised vaso-constrictor, ie. it causes the arteries to contract. The heart has to work harder to pump the blood around the body. If someone smokes twenty cigarettes a day, then his heart will beat an extra 10,000 beats in that 24 hours.

The effects of smoking are devastating for your heart. Nicotine causes raised blood pressure and an increased risk of bloods clots. Carbon monoxide reduces the blood's ability to absorb vital oxygen and is directly responsible for the development of cholesterol deposits on artery walls. The effect overall is an increased risk of heart attack and stroke.

Most smokers claim that a cigarette helps them to relax. If the heart is working so much harder because of the effects of nicotine, that claim becomes difficult to sustain, but what is worse is that, when cigarette smoke is introduced into the body, the organism reacts to being poisoned in the same way as it would if subjected to a horrifying experience. The automatic defence system becomes activated, and the whole body goes into what is known as 'fight or flight mode'.

This automatic response to danger is present in all creatures. It ensures that we are instantly prepared to use maximum strength and effort to either run from perceived danger or stop and fight. Our heart beats faster, and respiration increases to pump richly oxygenated blood to the major muscles and to the brain. Adrenaline and noradrenaline course through our system, and lactic acid is produced to maximise muscle power. The brain needs additional oxygen to heighten its ability to rationalise the situation and to react in the manner which best serves the need to survive the crisis. This process is highly visible in animals. The dog's hackles rise, and in humans the hairs on the back of the neck will stand up.

The whole body is in a high state of readiness for explosive maximum effort, and probably you have heard stories of how seemingly normal men and women are able to perform prodigious feats of strength and endurance in situations of great danger. An eight stone woman who lifts a car under which her son has become trapped when the jack slipped is just one example that springs to mind.

At the same time as this process of ensuring that the body's defence system is maximised to produce this seemingly superhuman strength, resources are diverted away from other areas that are less important. Systems which are not required are shut down to allow power to be available where it is most required.

The digestive system is hardly necessary when you are preparing to do battle or run from danger within the next few seconds, so it shuts down, and the ability to digest food and absorb the nutrients from it are dispensed with. Similarly blood supply to the extremities is reduced, and the immune system which will not be required to fight disease at this time, also shuts down.

What was that about, "It helps me to relax"?

When all around is chaos and unpredictable, we humans seek constancy and predictability and it can be seen that whatever else is happening and changing outside of our control and influence, "a cigarette stays the same". A cigarette is constant, it is predictable, it does provide at some level a sense of constancy and in this way can become a very potent influence, and therein lies the power of the habit.(Allen 1997)

There is an explanation. An element which is part of our survival instinct is the need to be comfortable. We do not like to feel cold, wet or hungry. I certainly do not appreciate any form of pain and will admit to being a complete wimp! The craving that is experienced as the subconscious delivers its message demanding that the nicotine levels be replenished is in no way something that can be described as pleasant. It is uncomfortable, and when we experience discomfort it does not improve our state of mind. Restlessness, anxiety and irritability are some of the emotional responses that are equated with discomfort. A cigarette satisfies the craving and so diminishes the discomfort, and therein is created the illusion that cigarettes promote a feeling of relaxation.

In normal circumstances, when the period of danger is over, the battle won or our escape made, the subconscious will relax its state of awareness and normal service will resume. This is the direct opposite of the 'fight or flight' response and is known as the 'relaxation' response. Now the heart beat returns to its normal level, as does respiration, and those functions which were temporarily shut down are brought back on line, and everything is fine again.

If we continue to smoke. The body is under constant assault, and the perception of danger is constant and unrelenting. The 'fight or flight' state that we have identified is still at a heightened state of readiness with all of those power diversions in operation: heart rate increased, respiration increased, adrenaline, noradrenaline and lactic acid production at full flow, digestive and immune systems suppressed. But, if we continue to smoke, the enzymes produced are not used in their intended fashion but remain in the tissues as toxins. Now we have a problem.

If a smoker cannot digest his food and absorb the nutrients from it efficiently because the digestive system has been suppressed, it is small wonder that smokers are so susceptible to health problems and suffer particularly from so many digestive upsets ranging from constipation to ulcers and cancers.

We need our immune system. We need it to fight with all its vigour to ensure that we have the maximum protection from the assaults on our health from so many quarters. Its function of seeking out and destroying invading organisms keeps us well protected from so many diseases that can kill and destroy our quality of life. It is at work constantly repairing the ravages of just being alive.

Cancer is the bogeyman of smoking. The main strategy of many smokers to diminish the possible threat to their health is dissociate themselves from it. "Cancer will not happen to me. It happens to other people." Even though we know that that is completely divorced from the truth, this perception serves to ensure that the smoking habit continues, as the 'smoker' part of the subconscious feeds this and other complete fallacies to the conscious mind to ensure the continued 'beneficial' supply of nicotine.

Cancer is a condition which is latent in everyone. It does not manifest itself in all of us, and indeed the majority live through life without this problem. It begins when the cell reproduction function which is controlled by the subconscious becomes corrupted and runs out of control. It is the immune system which protects us from this dreaded condition. A smoker's immune system is suppressed because of the permanent invocation of the fight or flight response, and this must surely be a major factor as to why smokers are much more susceptible to cancers that non smokers. The belief that smoking is responsible just for cancer of the lungs has to be discounted. True, lung cancer is sadly prevalent in smokers, but then this is the main avenue for the assault on the body perpetrated through smoking.

Smokers are at risk from cancer of the mouth, the tongue, the larynx, the kidneys, the liver, the prostate, the bladder, the testicles, the cervix, the womb and ovaries, the stomach and the colon, skin cancer, cancer of the oesophagus and cancer of the pancreas. In fact the incidence of any form of cancer that you can think of will be greatly increased.

The lungs

When we smoke, we inhale, drawing the gases produced by the burning tobacco into our lungs, gases full of chemicals and poisons.

The airways that conduct the inhaled air into the lungs are covered with fine hair-like projections called cilia. It is the function of the cilia to provide a defence against the ingress into the lungs of particles of dust and foreign matter.

An offending object will brush against the cilia, which are then activated to propel the foreign matter upwards again towards the mouth. The lungs and airways go into spasm as the delicate tissues of the linings are irritated and force air out in a violent explosion that is a cough. This reaction is designed to expel the foreign matter and prevent its passage down into the delicate inner chambers of the lungs where the vital interchange of gases is implemented. Oxygen is absorbed into the blood and carbon dioxide extracted and then expelled with exhalation.

Thick sticky tar in the cigarette smoke coats the tiny cilia causing them to become brittle, to lie flat against the walls of the airways, or to break off. They are thus unable to carry out their function so that the foreign particles are able to pass into the lungs where they accumulate. There is no way out. You may have seen pictures of lungs that have been removed from the cadavers of smokers showing the accumulation of soot and detritus from years of smoking. Not a pretty sight.

As the detritus accumulates the capacity of the lungs is reduced, and with that the ability to oxygenate the blood is also diminished. The mucus lining of the lungs that facilitates the chemical interaction necessary for the absorption of oxygen and the extraction of carbon dioxide becomes corrupted and its chemical composition changed. Its function impaired, the lungs produce more mucus in an attempt to correct the situation and so the lungs fill up with fluid. Here are the beginnings of chest diseases, the breathlessness and the horror of emphysema. As the lining of the bronchi are inflamed so begins the dreaded smoker's cough and because the bronchi are weakened so the smoker becomes more susceptible to recurring bronchial infections. Smokers are ten times more likely to contract lung cancer and emphysema than non-smokers.

The necessity of a good oxygen supply now requires the lungs with their reduced capacity to work harder to draw in enough air. This is the explanation for the gasping wheeze that is associated with long-term smoking. The ability to engage in any physical activity is adversely affected as the lungs begin to lose their ability to oxygenate the blood sufficiently to fuel the muscles for the extra activity. The smoker takes the lift or the escalator rather than use the stairs. That 'smoker' part of the subconscious will ensure that we get the message not to use the stairs. (*dissociative response)*

The kidneys and liver

The kidneys and the liver have the function of filtering out the waste matter in the body and excreting them. Due to the massive increase in poisons and toxins introduced through tobacco smoke, these organs need to work at a greatly increased rate in their attempt to clean the blood of the huge amounts of impurities.

The carcinogenic materials that are present in cigarettes pass of course through both these organs, increasing the likelihood that cancer will strike here. Kidney and liver failure is an increased risk that comes with smoking.

Gangrene

Every organ, every cell of our bodies, requires a good supply of nutrient-rich oxygenated blood. Without oxygen, tissues die. The effects of nicotine contract the arteries, the effects of carbon monoxide rob the blood of oxygen. The ability of the lungs to oxygenate the blood becomes progressive poorer, and the constant invocation of the fight or flight syndrome causes the blood supply to the extremities to be restricted. The immune system is repressed and struggles to cope with the constant ravages that are being inflicted on the body. Without oxygen, tissues die! Mortification of the flesh sets in: gangrene. To save a person's life, the surgeon has no option but to removes a leg, perhaps both. What is the quality of life now?

Sexual concern

Smoking attacks the very building blocks of life, the DNA. It attacks the eggs in the ovaries and it destroys sperm, reducing the count to levels where the chance of fathering healthy children is reduced and the danger of damage to the foetus is increased.

Sexual potency of smokers decreases more rapidly with age than that of non smokers, and similarly the incidence of impotence is also more prevalent. Smoking increases the ageing process, and a 50-year-old smoker is as old physically as a 70 year old non-smoker.

Women who smoke during pregnancy are poisoning and depriving their baby of oxygen whilst it is growing in the womb. The growing life inside the mother is reliant on a supply of nutrient-rich, well oxygenated blood in order to grow to be healthy. Babies born to women who smoke are generally smaller and are more susceptible to respiratory infections. Their development is slower and they do not do as well at school as children who are born to non-smoking parents.

Any mother who deliberately laced her child's food with arsenic and hydrogen cyanide, or fed nicotine to that infant, would be adjudged some sort of monster and guilty at the least of child abuse, if not murder. For a woman to carry a child through pregnancy with full knowledge that her smoking habit is damaging her baby, that she is depriving that child of oxygen and feeding it lethal poisons, has to place her in a position whereby she could be adjudged guilty of pre-natal child abuse.

The incidence of placenta separation is much higher in mothers who smoke, and the figures for miscarriage tell their own sad story, and a child born to a smoker is born addicted to nicotine and will be less content than a child who has been spared that fate.

High blood pressure is a well known risk that women face while carrying a child so, as smoking raises blood pressure, it is not a positive start to a pregnancy if the mother smokes.

With our bodies we enjoy the good things that life has to offer, and sexual relations play a huge part in the interaction between us. It is one of the joys of life, and the importance cannot be underestimated. To be a good lover it is necessary that we are the best and healthiest that we can be but how can we give of our best in that way unless we ensure that we look after our health, giving ourselves the best chance of remaining fit and virile. Smoking hardly achieves that!

A non-smoker is aware of some things that a smoker is not aware of. One of these is his ability to detect the smell of stale tobacco the instant a smoker comes into olfactory range. That smell permeates everything, hair, clothing, furnishings, and a smoker's breath can be very unpleasant.

Smokers are not welcome in many places now. Theatres, restaurants, buses, trains and planes all seek to ban smokers from their facilities. A smoker inhales just fifteen percent of the smoke from his cigarette, while the rest goes into the atmosphere so that others are subjected to passive smoking, without choice and may even find their clothes and hair also tainted with the smell.

Research in the USA during 1995 revealed that one carcinogen that exists only in tobacco smoke can be detected in the urine of non-smokers after exposure of just 90 minutes to conditions which are typical of a smoke filled room. In 1988 434,000 early deaths were attributed to the effects of smoking. 30,000 of these deaths were passive smoking related. If you are a parent and you smoke, then your children are 'passive smokers'. They will suffer an increased risk of asthma and other respiratory conditions.

British medical research shows that, in a study of male doctors who smoked between 1951–1994, the death rate in middle age was three times higher than those who never smoked. Approximately 50% of smokers die from causes which relate directly to their smoking.

Each time a smoker lights up a cigarette, that part of his subconscious mind that still tries to warn him about the dangers is overpowered by the part that wants to keep him smoking. There is usually a pang of guilt present but unfortunately ignored.

At least now filters are fitted to many brands of cigarettes in an attempt to filter out some of the poisons so some smokers will live just a little longer. However, statistically each cigarette reduces life expectancy by six minutes.

It seems incredible that our smoker, faced with all these facts, nevertheless continue to smoke. These facts will be accepted at a conscious level, but we need to effect changes at the subconscious level for him to view the situation differently. The subconscious smoker is determined not to alter what it considers to be necessary for survival. In some cases, of course, with sheer effort of will, a smoker will give up, but those who come to the therapist's office recognise a need in themselves for help in achieving their goal.

It may be that the need is for a formalised ceremony, ie. the therapy session, that will mark the end of one era and the beginning of a new one.

I would submit that there are those for whom the therapy session is just a confirmation of the decision already made and that they have indeed already achieved their non-smoking status before they reach the office. But they have identified a need within themselves for the formal ceremonial that is the therapy session. We as therapists should be careful here and be aware of the forces that have maintained the client's smoking habit and aware of the nature of the subconscious "part" to use every trick in the book to carry out its purpose. *In this initial period when you are seeking to consolidate changes in you behaviour associated with ceasing to smoke there may be a voice in your head which says, "It's OK to have a cigarette, just one won't hurt you."(Citrenbaum, King & Cohen 1985)*

The therapist must conduct the therapy with much expertise, having gained information as to the nature of the clients addiction, hopes, fears and aspirations. And it is now that I address the content of the therapy session with regard to the nature and style of effective interventions with due consideration of the nature of the subconscious forces that we are seeking to change.

The information so far provided in these pages will enable the therapist to dissect the client's smoking habit, and confront, with clarity and irrefutable facts, all the myths and misconceptions which the client is likely to put forward.

As therapists we present ourselves as experts in what we do, so it is necessary to be well informed about the dangers we are seeking to help our client avoid.

With the client formally hypnotised there are a number of approaches that we can use to deliver the interventions that are designed to effect the changes that will help him to achieve the aim of the therapy.

In order to determine the most effective approaches, we will have been using our powers of observation during the time we have thus far spent with the client. There is so much that we can learn from being an acute observer. It may be that the manner in which a person conducts himself will give us a clue. A person with a military background, for example, will conduct himself in a manner which is precise and ordered, his bearing in accordance with the conditioning that we recognise as being military.

Perhaps this person will respond to a very direct approach. Accustomed to taking orders from his superiors, he may well see the therapist as a figure of authority. "You will not smoke" is an order that must be obeyed. Every client brings with him much information that the observant therapist can identify and use.

I remember well a young man of 24 years who came to see me for smoking cessation. He was a Royal Marine Commando and very proud of the elite body to which he belonged. In the preamble it was established that he placed great store on team-work and being able to rely on his comrades in arms and to have them confident of relying on him.

I asked him to visualise a scene where he was on parade with his company. I told him that he was to address the parade and explain to his comrades that he would no longer be part of the team. He had been declared unfit because of his smoking habit and was therefore no longer eligible to be a Royal Marine Commando. The effect of this strategy was dramatic. This tough marine who had seen action in the Falklands was in tears and completely distraught.

I then asked him to access the part that had been responsible for his smoking habit and addressed the matter of what smoking had achieved for him. It helped when bored, was the answer. The reframing approach was the obvious strategy to use as I asked him if he found the observation duties that he had told me about earlier to be boring. He had been obliged to hide and observe enemy positions for considerable periods of time. He said that it was cold and wet and "balls aching". I asked him if he had found his smoking to be a help at that time. "No way! I did not want to give my position away." "So not smoking perhaps saved your life at that time?" He agreed with me that to smoke would have been suicidal.

"So what would you consider a good way to alleviate boredom and ensure that you remain healthy and fit that is more beneficial than smoking?"

This is of course just one example of many, and the direction taken was dictated by the unique individual situation. It is most important for the therapist to be ever ready to step off the well worn path and allow his/her own subconscious instincts to dictate the direction in which the therapy should proceed.

"You will be intensely aware of the enemy that is tobacco, no longer camouflaged, his position detected and clearly marked. You are aware of the danger to health and life that smoking represents, aware of your duty to ensure that all is done to preserve your ability to carry through your duty. You have no desire or need to smoke."

The use of metaphors to imbed suggestions is more effective as the message in a story is assimilated at a subconscious level.

A story does not need to be truthful or factual; it is simply a vehicle for the message that we wish to convey, and everyone loves stories. There is a beneficial effect for the client. Each of us will relate the story to our own experiences, and in this way beneficial changes can occur in our lives.

As we formulate our approach to therapy, it is necessary to consider other factors that have been at work to keep the smoker smoking. These include strategies that his subconscious has employed to justify his continued smoking.

The message on the pack of cigarettes says, "Smoking can seriously damage health". Each time a smoker reaches for the pack he is aware of the message, but still lights up, disregarding what should be sufficient warning to prevent him. If we see a sign on the beach that reads, "Dangerous currents. Do not swim", does that not ensure that our common sense will prevent us from taking the risk?

What we are seeing here is the subconscious strategy of dissociation, or denial – The "it won't happen to me" syndrome. Though the smoker is consciously aware of all of the dangers to his health and even perhaps despite warnings from his doctor, his subconscious tells him that he will be fine, or that just one cigarette will not hurt. It may even give the message that it's too late now, or that it doesn't matter, or that the doctor is just trying to scare him.

How often have I heard the story, "What smell? I can't smell anything or "I don't smoke many", and the person telling me that is sure he is telling the truth. To him each cigarette smoked is "just one that won't hurt". Previous cigarettes have been conveniently forgotten and discounted. Reality is thus distorted and truth denied as the "smoker" part continues its task with great ingenuity and invention.

I remember a story told to me by a fellow hypnotherapist who, whilst attending the funeral of an old friend, was drawn into conversation with a man who chain smoked his way through the service and the internment.

The therapist remarked in a kindly fashion that the amount of cigarettes being smoked must be costing a fortune. The smoker replied that he needed the cigarettes to help him through the anxious time of losing his father whose funeral it was. He claimed that the cigarettes calmed him. His father had died from lung cancer a few years after losing a leg to the surgeon's knife, all attributed to his smoking.

His mother who was also at the funeral of her husband was suffering from arteriosclerosis and the beginnings of emphysema, and yet she too demonstrated how much she needed her nicotine fix. The powerful urge to continue smoking certainly demands our respect in its ability to completely ignore such dire warnings.

What must the 'subconscious smoker' part be telling a mother which so powerfully ensures her continuing to smoke and poisoning her unborn baby? How does she dissociate from the truth that is so apparent? It does not fall within the realm of rationality because it is irrational. The secondary gains even though completely non-beneficial are able to override the factual evidence.

"Don't bore me with facts. I have made up my mind."

Maladaprive coping mechanisms that are indicative of deep seated emotional problems may need to be addressed before the client is even accepted for smoking cessation therapy. To a great degree the success of therapy depends on the screening of clients by the therapist and the rejection of those who really are not at a point in their life where there is a reasonable chance of success.

The client who is also a heavy drinker has a diminished chance of success in quitting smoking because of the effect of alcohol in lowering inhibition. I would suggest that both situations need to be addressed together. The client needs to understand that, if he wishes to stop smoking, his drinking must be reduced to a level that will allow for a greater chance of success.

This may seem a little harsh to some therapists who are just beginning in practice and who wish to see as many clients as possible. However it will benefit the therapist if those who are not suitable for therapy are screened out as they will appreciate this honesty and professionalism. Very often the client will accept the decision and seek help for the underlying problem, and when this has been resolved this will lead to an opportunity to help them successfully to give up the smoking which has been part of their maladaptive coping mechanism.

The smoker who declares the right to do what he wants with his own body is a typical example of how powerful denial can prove. He will steadfastly insist that smoking is one of his life pleasures and that there can be no reason to listen to the killjoys who just want to control him. He will demand the right to smoke on trains and planes, in restaurants and cinemas etc., in a crusading manner bordering on the obsessive.

What he is in fact saying, prompted by his own subconscious smoking mind, is that he cannot do without the pleasure that is perceived. The truth is that he cannot cope with the uncomfortable consequences of ceasing to appease his own 'subconscious smoker' which will make him feel so uncomfortable through the cravings and withdrawal effects that it can create. The opposite to pain and distress is pleasure and calm security, regardless of the reality of the consequences which are dealt with through dissociation tactics.

The result is an overblown often vehement defence of the habit. *Methinks he doth protest too much (William Shakespeare, The Merchant of Venice)*

The 'subconscious smoker', with its back to the wall, is going to use every trick in its armoury to provide both physical need and then justification for the smoker, now trying so hard to quit, to continue. It cannot be denied that, in order to beat the habit, the gauntlet of withdrawal symptoms will have to be run. The voice will say something like, "Go on. Just one will help you to feel better so that you can really make the effort later", or "Just one will not hurt. After all you have managed to stop for four days now and that proves that you can stop when you want to" or "It's easy to stop, but right at this moment, there is no need for you to prove it, and nobody will know".

There is a school of thought that says to stop smoking abruptly is the wrong way to tackle this problem, that it is far better to taper off slowly and then eventually stop. I cannot agree with this at all. This just prolongs the period of discomfort. If the "subconscious smoker" is getting less than it needs, then it will increase its demands as the levels of nicotine decrease.

The smoker who tries a smaller or lower strength brand of cigarette, only to find that he needs to smoke more cigarettes than before, proves this. The demands for nicotine will remain at the same level, thus an increased consumption is likely to be required in order to satisfy the same craving.

Athletes do not smoke. The demands for peak physical performance have completely negated the myth that the body can still function optimally when subjected to abuse.

Smokers become out of breath when indulging in physical exercise and, in order to ensure that they are not reminded of this, they modify their involvement and do not generally indulge in those activities which demand a fully functioning respiratory system. Smokers do not take the stairs, they take the elevator, for the same reason.

This can be seen as a learned response to an anticipated unpleasant experience.

I well remember one man in his early thirties telling me that he had smoked since the age of thirteen years and felt absolutely fine. I explained to him that he was not in any position to judge whether or not he was in fact fine, as he had no experience of getting older without the effects of his smoking habit. If you haven't had it, you can hardly miss it. It had never occurred to him to consider his own situation in that way.

Associations

In the same way as the 'subconscious smoker' denies that which does not suit its purpose, it also uses prompts to ensure that the habit continues. We form habits through repetition which then becomes a process of association. We associate a hammer with a nail, bread with butter, and bat with ball. These are useful associates and cannot be seen as dangerous in any way. Our subconscious employs this technique in order that we can put things into logical frameworks.

But the 'subconscious smoker' utilises this simple device to much more sinister ends. It tells our smoker, "The car will not start without a cigarette" or "A meal is not complete without a cigarette". A pint of beer can be linked to a cigarette. It can be interesting to watch a smoker who has just finished a meal. The plate is pushed away, and a glazed look comes over his face as he goes into a trance during which a packet of cigarettes is pulled from his pocket, a cigarette is placed in the mouth and then lit. There is no conscious awareness of the whole of this process: it is purely subconscious.

The telephone is a favourite. Many people do not have the ability to answer a telephone unless they have a cigarette. Each time the phone rings the 'subconscious smoker' is saying, "It's time for a cigarette". It delivers the same message when the call is outgoing: the telephone system is useless without that most integral of components.

You will not put on weight if you smoke. Okay, tobacco does suppress the appetite. Its effects suppress the whole of the digestive system. The truth is, of course, that if you eat more than you need you will put on weight as a natural consequence. An element of paranoia can creep into the proceedings, and a well-timed remark as to any weight gain will provide a powerful incentive for the reformed smoker to take up the habit again. Smoking damages our health and kills us much more effectively than food. Smokers who are aiming to quit should be aware of the need for balanced nutrition.

Because people drink and smoke at parties, the association with having a good time and smoking is easily established. It really is amazing to me that people who have stopped smoking will come to me with the story, "I was at this party, and a group of my friends were having a whale of a time, cracking jokes, drinking and smoking. I felt really left out of things because I was not smoking with them".

The smoking was in this situation a means of establishing a bond between friends, and the giving of a cigarette to a friend conveys acceptance as one of the group. Suddenly that bonding element is no longer present, and the 'subconscious smoker' sees another opportunity to make our reformed smoker feel bad. "You will feel so much more comfortable when you are joining in with your friends. Just one won't hurt, and you can stop again tomorrow". Craftier than a barrel of monkeys and more dangerous than a rattlesnake is the true nature of that friendly enemy!

How is it that the hands on the ends of your arms can feel so clumsy and obtrusive? A cigarette gives you something to do with your hands. So why not a pen, a rubber ball or a haddock? The whole idea of a cigarette as a prop to help with confidence is nonsense and can easily be seen as just that, but the 'subconscious smoker' has its way of delivering such nonsense in a manner that has one purpose in mind, to maintain the smoking habit and thereby its supply of nicotine.

Formatting the therapy session

I am not shy of using scripted material in the correct context. It is useful to have at hand a form of words that can be used to address various therapeutic goals. The key is adaptation and utilisation. I have with me at all times a special book of plastic loose pockets into which I slip many carefully worded pieces to which I can refer as required. If I wish to create a particular visualisation, it is easy to flip to that page and then, using the frame of the script, adapt it to my particular client. It ensures that the semantics employed are those which have been considered.

In the following section I will work through a session with a client. This session is actually composed of an amalgamation of many. With the purpose of demonstrating to the best effect the use of various strategies and techniques.

The main elements of reframing, of imbedded and of direct suggestion coupled with visualisations and suggested experience, are all incorporated in this session. Whilst I expect that readers of this work will be experienced in the induction of hypnotic trance, I will include an induction which is taken from my earlier book, *Scripts and Strategies in Hypnotherapy*.

Smoking Questionnaire

I include for guidance a copy of the questionnaire that I normally use with my clients. I suggest that you leave your client alone for about ten minutes to ensure that each question does not provoke a time consuming verbalisation of his experience. Once completed, you, the therapist, can then choose which elements of the questionnaire to expand upon, remaining in control of the session. To a significant degree, the questionnaire is useful in that it does help to concentrate the thoughts of the client on what is important.

Name: ____

Age: ________ Marital status: ___________________________

Occupation: ____

Is your work stressful? No ❑ Moderately ❑ Very ❑

Partner's name: _____________________________________

Age: ________ Children: ________

Do any others in your family smoke? Yes ❑ No ❑

How many cigarettes do you smoke in a day? _____

At what age did you start smoking? _____

Why did you start? Peer pressure ❑
Rebel against authority ❑
To appear more adult ❑
Other: ______________________________

What do you get from smoking? It relaxes me ❑
It helps me to concentrate ❑
It's an excuse for a break ❑
It give me a confidence boost ❑
It's a prop ❑
Other: ____________________

When do you smoke? On waking ❑
At breakfast ❑
With tea/coffee ❑
After meals ❑
Driving ❑
On the phone ❑
At work ❑
In bed ❑
Other: ______________________________

What frightens you about smoking? ______________________

____

Do you know someone who has died from a smoking related disease? Yes ❑ No ❑

Do you know someone who is ill now? Yes ❑ No ❑

What is important to you? ___________________________

____

Who are you important to? Why? _______________________

____

Has your doctor mentioned your smoking? Yes ❑ No ❑

Have you had any worrying symptoms? Yes ❑ No ❑

Do you have any health problems? Heart problems ❑
High blood pressure ❑
Diabetes ❑
Asthma ❑
Ulcers ❑
Other ❑

How long do you want to live? _____ Why?____________________

____

Who is responsible for your health? ____________________________

What will you be able to do as a non-smoker that you could not do before?

____

____

What will you do with the money that you save? ________________

____

Do you really wish to commit yourself to stopping smoking?
Yes ❑
No ❑

What is stopping you? ______________________________________

____

Observations: ____

____

____

____

____

Experience Induction

This induction is appropriate for anxious clients. Contraindication: clients who have a fear of water.

(Achieve Eye Closure)

Now you are resting comfortably there listening to the sound of my voice **here**, with your eyes closed comfortably, and you can be aware of your eyes and of how you are in control ... and how you could open them should you wish … and that's fine, because I really wouldn't want you to not go into hypnosis too quickly. I would prefer that you discover how much easier it is … simply to allow events to occur in their own time and in their own way ... and as you allow that feeling to continue in a shoulder ... a leg ... a hand … as you continue to listen to the sound of my voice ... the sounds that surround you ... the ticking of the clock perhaps or the distant murmur of traffic ... paying close attention now to those feelings ... those changes as they occur as you wonder at your own ability to let go completely and drift into a trance, while your conscious mind has already begun to drift off somewhere else ... allowing your body to relax and your mind to relax … without knowing at all how much more comfortable and **relaxed** you can become.

I wonder if you can remember now those experiences of drifting off whilst sitting comfortably watching television … so engrossed in the story line ... listening to the voices as your eyes closed … to rest quietly for a moment in time … hearing the music … those words spoken … in that quiet and **relaxed** way , when a word or a sound brings to mind a particular memory ... and you drift into that memory ... dream away for a time … coming back to the words again ... until the words and the music become a soothing murmur ... a relaxing sound ... heard only in the background of the mind ... like a conversation overheard … a peaceful and quiet time … and the subconscious of your mind continues to hear all that is important to you ... whilst your conscious mind drifts off to another place without really noticing that there is no need for you to make the effort to try, to hear ... or to understand everything that is said or not said **here**, as you rest so quietly, **there**. You really have known all along how much easier it is to learn when you are so **relaxed** ... though I wouldn't want you to relax too quickly at first ... I would prefer that you discover now how much easier it is to recognise the small changes ... tiny changes ... almost imperceptible changes ... happening in your breathing ... and in your pulserate ... how quiet and comfortable you have become as that feeling of security relaxes you even deeper than before. Your unconscious may choose to relax just one of your fingers before it continues to relax one of your thumbs ... or perhaps it will discover that your wrist will be a handier place to begin relaxing, but the conscious part of your mind can enjoy being curious about exactly where those feelings will begin.

And now *(client's name)* please consider a stone being skipped across the clear calm surface of a pond ... The stone skips once ... twice ... three times and more ... and each time the intervals become shorter as it loses momentum ... slowing ... down more and more ... as it strikes the surface. The peace and tranquillity is disturbed. The water flows in ripples that spread out in perfect rings ... but then the stone can skip no more ... All momentum is dissipated, its power lost ... and so it slips quietly down beneath the surface, gently floating down ... past the creatures that live here ... drifting down ... gently ... quietly ... past the water plants ... and nothing is disturbed as it finally comes to rest there ... still now on the bottom of the tranquil pool ... and on the surface ... even the ripples become quieter as they spread in ever increasing circles ... eventually to disappear entirely as the surface becomes calm again and you can take the opportunity to quietly reflect upon those problems as you recognise now that ability that is yours ... to relax ... to let go of tension ... anxiety ... aware now of your ability to see things in a different way ... and to accept those things that seem to be one thing and then turn out to be something else entirely ... and then the difficulty and ease that can be your experience of telling the difference between souls and soles ... sun and son ... bear and bare ... changing old beliefs ... recognising new capabilities and capacities ... learning new ways of doing things.

I wonder now if you can allow those feelings to continue the same or to deepen even more now as you try to remember all those things

I have said here … about that pool there … that television … that stone that drifted down slowly … even as you drift with you own thoughts … and enjoy allowing that pleasant and comfortable experience of heaviness of arms, of legs … to continue there now as I continue to talk to you … each word that I speak … relaxing you deeper still.

(You can judge at this point whether you need to use a deepener script or continue with the session as you have planned.)

The Hypno-Therapeutic Session

The following format represents a framework within which to work. I use information gathered from the client, along with various techniques and strategies to implement the therapeutic changes necessary for a successful outcome for the client. It is important to stress that this forms only a framework: aversion techniques are fine and are extremely effective with some clients, but not all. Great consideration must therefore be given to the client's attitude and feelings so as to ensure that the session is effective without being offensive or causing undue stress.

That's fine *(client's name)* ... You are doing so well ... and perhaps you can recognise just how comfortable you can feel as each breath that you take allows you to drift even deeper into trance ...You have co-operated so well with me, and it really is a pleasure to work with someone such as you who can believe that the success of your therapy will be assured as you continue to listen to the sound of my voice and those things which are so important to you.

It can be a relaxing experience to discover that you have been aware all along that you know of the real reason for your smoking. ... It is that addiction to nicotine that seemed so strong yet now is overpowered by your commitment and your total determination as you cast off the need and the desire for all tobacco products ... All that is left is a habit problem ... You have no need or desire to smoke ... you know that ... so it will be easy ... It is now you versus tobacco and you will easily win because you are stronger than any habit created by your own mind could possibly be.

You have continued to smoke ... because you have been doing it unconsciously ... but from this moment forward you will be aware of every moment of your smoking ... The instant that you reach for a cigarette you will be intensely aware of that cigarette, and if you begin to smoke it you will be aware of all the good reasons for giving it up and all the negative and painful consequences of your smoking.

You will become disgusted with the smell and the foul taste that your subconscious will remind you of ... as it reminds you now ... that taste and noxious smell ... so long ignored and now so powerful as not to be ignored or denied. When you are fully aware of your smoking ... it is no longer an unconscious habit; you are doing it on purpose and that is not the same.

You already have no need or desire to continue smoking ... this you know ... so stopping smoking will be easy ... It will be effortless.

There will be no struggle with will power ... no guilt of smoking ... Your new and powerful awareness may make you bored with smoking ... disgusted and annoyed ... You will have no desire or need to smoke at all.

That foul taste and smell will remind you of all of the good and healthy reasons for giving it up and you will find it easy to give up those things that you do not like ... **You do not like to smoke and so you are giving it up.** ...You are giving it up **now** ... not tomorrow ... not next week but right now as of this second you are giving up all the pain and the guilt of all the negative aspects of smoking ... You now choose life ... good health and happiness and you have no need or desire for tobacco products.

Now *(client's name)* I can accept that there is a subconscious part of you that wants to smoke and that part has my sincere respect ... It can appear so powerful ... and despite the fact that you want to stop smoking ... It will quit only when it is ready to do so.

Reframe

I want you now to go deep inside your own mind and as you go deeper with every breath ... I wonder how quickly you can in the next minute ... experience that part of you that I will call your 'subconscious smoker' which has been responsible for your smoking.

Perhaps you can ask your subconscious to allow me to be aware that it is allowing you that experience by lifting the index finger of your right hand. *(Touch finger ... ideomotor response)*

Of course ... I appreciate that this co-operation may be something that it will wish to keep private and that is fine ... Please just continue with that understanding ... I do not know just how you will experience that 'smoker part' of you that believes that you need to smoke ... or what special language will allow you to enjoy that special communication with that part in some way that is safe and comfortable to be experienced by your conscious mind ... as I ask you *(client's name)* to seek the answers to some important questions that you need to understand in order to achieve your goal.

As you listen to my voice ... concentrate intently on that internal communication that becomes so clear as you recognise now that part of you has been keeping you smoking because of some benefits or pay-offs ... I would like you now to ask your 'smoker part' to tell you now of the pay-offs and benefits of your smoking. I understand that the behaviour of that 'smoker part' has caused you to suffer negative and unhealthy consequences ... but I want to suggest that you now re-assess your understanding of your smoking to realise that the intention of your 'smoker part' has been to help you or to benefit you in some way.

Now *(client's name)* ... please take some special time and go deep inside to your inner mind and become aware of the pay-offs and benefits that are associated with your smoking.

Has smoking helped you to get something that some part of you wanted? ... perhaps attention from family or friends?

Has smoking helped you to avoid something that a part of you would find painful or uncomfortable? ... perhaps intimacy? ... Again I am asking you to continue with the assumption that your 'inner smoker' has continued up to now because it has helped you or benefited you in some way ... so ... please become aware if it is comfortable and safe for you to have this awareness of how your smoking has helped you.

(In your notes there may well be something specific that you have observed that can be now suggested for consideration)

Now keeping these pay-offs and benefits in mind ... I want to suggest to you *(client's name)* that there are alternative ways of experiencing or of perceiving that can provide you with all of those pay-offs and benefits that smoking has provided for you in the past ... but be so much healthier for you.

Now *(client's name)* ... please take some special time and go into your mind.

As you go deep inside I would like you to allow that part of you which is so creative ... that can provide solutions to problems with your best interests paramount ... to construct some alternative behaviours that you can easily substitute for your smoking that will provide all of those pay-offs and benefits that smoking has provided for you in the past.

I want you to take all the time you need within the next two minutes to check with that part of you and all other parts of you that these new alternatives seem acceptable and are seen to be acceptable ... sound acceptable and feel acceptable to that part and to all parts of you ...

If you experience anything which appears to be a "No" signal such as increased tension or irritability in response to your new alternatives ... then that is okay ... you will need to go back inside your mind perhaps even further to where acceptable new alternatives can be generated ... Perhaps you may need to take into account some benefits or pay-offs that you were not aware of before.

If your alternatives are okay ... then you can proceed with what we call 'future pacing'.

Please go back into your inner mind again and allow your imagination to show you yourself in those places ... those times and those situations where you have smoked in the past ... See yourself now aware of and utilising your new alternative patterns of behaviour that your creative mind has constructed for you.

See yourself on the phone ... not smoking ... finishing your meal ... not smoking ... driving your car ... not smoking. Imagine yourself in these and all other contexts where you used to smoke ... using all your new and healthier alternatives.

If you experience any difficulty ... it may be necessary for you to go back and generate more suitable alternatives. Perhaps you need to take into account some future context that you have just become aware of.

If you have successfully imagined future contexts using your new alternatives ... then you have successfully completed this re-framing process.

I would like to suggest that you now thank that part of you for its beneficial communication and express your appreciation for the healthy work that has been done as I too express my appreciation.

I can understand that you may not be consciously aware of the work that has taken place but you can know that your subconscious is fully aware and may even have taken the opportunity to do some work for you on other habit problems that you may have and you will be pleasantly surprised when you discover that you find it so easy to conquer other habits.

I want to congratulate you *(client's name)* ... on the excellent work you have done ... and now as you listen to my voice ... you can find that you can concentrate on that sound ... concentrating to a pin-point as all other sounds fade into insignificance ... As you now allow yourself to enjoy the peace and tranquillity of that special place that is yours ... where you can be so **relaxed** you can recognise those signs of hypnosis ... heaviness of legs ... of arms ... a feeling of calm and of security.

You will forget about cigarettes altogether ... You have no need to buy them because you have no need to smoke them ... and so you will enjoy the special things that the money saved will provide for you. (*Give example e.g. a holiday that he may have mentioned)* You have given up all the things that you don't want ... and you look forward to all those things that you do want. You know that you want to stop smoking and you know why. That reason forms clearly in your mind and should you ever through momentary lapse or childish impulse ... ever put a cigarette to your lips again ... your subconscious will provide you with a disgusting and powerful reminder of the harm to health ... the powerful stench and the nauseating taste of stale tobacco ... not to be ignored or denied. You will be aware of a powerful compulsion to break cigarettes in two and scatter the tobacco to the wind.

If ever you accept an offered cigarette ... then you will break that cigarette in two and it will remind you of all the bad things you are giving up and of the good things that are in store for you as a natural non-smoker.

Self-hypnosis tuition

As you are so **relaxed** and so comfortable now ... feeling so very positive about your success in stopping smoking ... I want to teach you self-hypnosis that you can use any time that you need to or want to.

In a moment I am going to have you open your eyes and then make a tight fist with your right hand or your left hand ... Whichever you choose is fine ... I want you then to count from ten backwards to zero as you concentrate on the tightness of that hand ... With each count the tightness will loosen more and more and by the time or before you get to zero ... all of that tension will have disappeared and your eyes can close as you drift back to that comfortable state of hypnosis where you are right now.

Okay *(client's name)* ... open your eyes now ... Now make that fist with your right hand or your left hand and concentrate on that tightness ... Concentrate on the tension in that hand as you begin now to count backwards from ten to zero aware of that tension as it diminishes with each count ... Try to get all the way back to zero before that you find that all that tension has gone and your eyes close ... *(Wait until the eyes close)* That's right ... relaxing ... releasing just letting go completely ... drifting into that trance state ... where you really can go into your mind and ask that it does all those things that it can do for your highest good ... aware that there really is no need for you to make the effort to try to be aware of how it does those things for you ... or to remember any or all of what is said or not said here as you rest so quietly there ... *(Suggestion for amnesia)* That's good *(client's name)* ... You have all that you need ... patience ... determination and commitment to those things that are for your highest benefit ... You can just make that fist ... make that count ...

as you utilise your own ability to go into hypnosis ... You can utilise that ability to strengthen your resolve and your commitment as that person who has no desire and no need to smoke and you will, will you not? *(Await response)*

You are doing so well *(client's name)* ... It really is a pleasure to be able to work with someone who is so committed and who co-operates so very well with me.

I would like to ask you to ask your subconscious to help you now with an ability that you have to look forward in time ... that ability that you have to imagine just what it would be like if this happened or that did not happen ... I would like you to see yourself in a familiar place ... it could be your own front room ... in your garden ... it does not matter at all where as long as you also experience you being amongst all those people whom you love and who love you and rely on you to be there for them. Here in that place see your family. *(Give names of close family ... children etc.)* They are all here gathered from far and near ... They have come here because of what you have to tell them. *(Begin now to harden your voice)*

You have to tell them that despite all of the warnings from your doctor and those who want so much for you to stop smoking ... you have some very bad news. Hospital tests have shown that you have contracted cancer ... something that could never happen to you. You made the choice to ignore the good advice and the wishes of those who care so much for you and now this horrifying disease has progressed so quickly and is now so far advanced that there is little if anything that medical science can do for you ... Your days are numbered and perhaps you have just months to live ... Soon you will be gone, your life ended prematurely like so many before you ... I want you to tell them now ... and as you tell them this dreadful truth ... tell them just who is responsible ... watch their faces ... see the shock ... the disbelief ... the horror and then the grief and the anger too. An insidious habit has robbed you of your life and those who care for you and rely on you ... of that person who is so very special to them. *(Pause)* How do you feel?

(This utilisation of shock/aversion tactics can be specifically tailored to the person using the information that you have gained from your observations. The grandmother who is not allowed to hold her new born

grandson ... or the uncle or aunt who is asked to keep away from little Johnny whose asthma will be aggravated by the smell on their clothing and in their hair. I am sure that you can come up with some useful variations on this theme).

(Soften your voice now)

Those who love you and care so much for you will be pleased that you have made a commitment to yourself to quit immediately that destructive and foul habit ... taking for yourself that complete responsibility for your own health and your own life.

I wonder now just how good you can feel as you feel that growing expanding awareness of the importance and significance of the decision you have made and the commitment to take in full the responsibility for your own health, for your own life and happiness ... and you can feel justifiably proud of that achievement that is yours as your confidence in your ability to take charge of your own life ... to set that good example to those who look up to you and admire you ... and all of those things that are so important ... grows stronger and stronger with every day ... as you grow better and better and better with every moment of each new day of your life.

You are a **natural non-smoker. ...** You are pleased and proud to be the person that you are ... That positive image becomes complete and you accept yourself without question ... without condition as a natural non-smoker ... You find it difficult now to even remember to try to recall the feeling of wanting or needing or enjoying a cigarette ... the image is complete and has become an integral part of **you** making a deep ... vivid and **permanent** impression on your perfect subconscious mind ... You look to the future now ... calm ... confident ... optimistic as you eagerly anticipate all the good and positive things that are in store for you ... You realise that the past is past ... the habit ... the harm and the memory of smoking belong to the past and you firmly close the door to the past ... along with any doubts or fears ... guilt or self-limitations.

Looking always to the future ... each new day is a new step towards the realisation of your goals, your hopes and aspirations ... a new step toward the attainment of your highest and true potential.

In a few moments it will be time for you to return to full awareness bringing with you a feeling of balance and of calm confidence in your own capacities and capabilities ... a knowing that you have a special knowledge of all your special needs to eat wisely ... to exercise moderately and safely and to practise regularly your ability to use self-hypnosis and recognise the good counsel of your own inner mind ... your own wise inner advisor.

You recognise that there is no need at all for you to remember all these concepts ... They are now a vital and integral part of your inner mind that serves you in all things ... reflecting spontaneously and dynamically in your natural behaviour each of these ideas ... positive suggestions and ideas ... because they come from a fount of knowledge and self understanding deep within the very essence of the person that you are.

Trance termination.

Reasoned Intervention

Nothing is completely new, just revamped and sometimes improved. Recognising that a hammer is best used to drive in a nail as is a screwdriver to drive in a screw, is imperative. If all you have in your toolbox is a hammer, then everything can appear to be a nail. Sadly there are still some people out there who continue to trot out the same tired old techniques. A GP will continue to prescribe a particular drug for a recognised ailment, but for the GP it is good practice, as the condition he will be treating is usually specific and its course predictable.

As therapists, however, dealing with the symptoms produced by anxious and maladjusted subconscious processes, we do not have that luxury of specific diagnosis and treatment. There are no text-book cases for us, and a smoker is not just a smoker. He is a unique human being who for reasons of coping with elements of his life has established a perceived need to smoke.

It is because we are not always privy to the reasons that are the causative events that generate the presenting symptoms that I place so much value on the specific reframing technique developed by Richard Bandler and John Grinder, for the work of change may well continue unseen and unheard by us therapists but with undeniably beneficial effects as the client is guided to invoke the power of his own subconscious mind to achieve desired therapeutic change.

Whenever a client appears at a therapist's door, he comes with certain expectations. He may have been recommended to come by a friend who has successfully stopped smoking with the aid of hypnotherapy. "Go and see Roger Allen. I did and I haven't smoked since", may be what prompts him to make the telephone call to set up an appointment. It is not unreasonable to expect that, because he has been told that Roger Allen is the best, he will stop smoking as soon as Roger Allen has worked his magic.

There is a school of thought that tells us that we should not encourage these misconceptions about hypnosis or the "power" that we have to affect the lives and habits of people. I would venture this thought for consideration, **"If it works, why fix it"?**

Looking back through the annals of time we see so many examples of the ways in which the beliefs of people can manifest themselves. The shaman and the witch doctors have utilised the belief systems of their subjects with documented effect. To be precise, "If you believe it will work, then it will work". Another phrase that springs to mind is "self fulfilling prophecy".

I would not advocate deliberately creating an unrealistic expectation, but who of us can say that it is unrealistic if, armed with that belief, a client undergoes therapy and the desired result is achieved? Does it really matter?

So often I have found myself faced with a client who tells me that hypnosis is magic and will provide the solution to his problem. My immediate impulse is to educate this person, but over the years I have learned to carefully consider what is my role. Am I there to provide instruction in the truths and otherwise of hypnosis or am I there to utilise the material that my client is supplying me with? If the therapy is successful, is it because the client believes, and if not successful, then perhaps he did not believe enough? I can appear to be a nice guy, taking the time and the trouble to persuade this person that his perception is flawed and that the magical effect will just not happen. Have I reduced the chances of successful therapy by proving how well informed I am, or have I perhaps just massaged my own ego?

Much of the effectiveness of hypnotherapy has to be accepted as a placebo, but how much I do not know. Let us all accept that hypnosis is a potent tool in our efforts to effect therapeutic change and for whatever reason be grateful that it does work and that lives change, become more meaningful and problems can be resolved.

If the belief system of a client is flawed and as a result adversely affects the quality of that person's life then the changes that are necessary are not in education, but in changes of perception at a level where it can produce symptom erradication in a situation where that symptom is considered to be a maladjusted response that produces more harm than good. We know that all our smoker clients are consciously aware of the harm that they do to themselves and we are also aware that it is not just by educating them about the damage to their health that will help them to stop, but that reframing of their perceptions is what is necessary.

I find that the most common concern expressed has to do with "control". Can I, using hypnosis, take control of my client's mind? This question of course stems from misconceptions that are the result of stage shows where it really can appear that the hypnotist is controlling the minds of those who are his subjects.

With some basic training in the nature of and the value of hypnosis as a therapeutic tool, it will be realised that hypnosis is not something that we "do" to someone, but rather that he does in response to our suggestions. If he chooses to resist our suggestions, then hypnotic trance is not achieved. The hypnotist can only utilise the ability of the client to achieve a state that we term hypnotic trance with his compliance and co-operation.

I would usually answer the question, "Can you control my mind?", with something in the manner of, "My bank manager doesn't seem to think so!". The question is answered, but the final analysis is left to the client, and therefore the "magical expectation" aspect can still remain to serve a useful purpose.

We need to enlist the trust of our client as early in the proceedings as possible. This is vital to ensure his full co-operation when inducing trance and continuing with the therapy session.

"Now *(client's name)*, you may be concerned at your ability to go into trance. Well I would like you to know that you do have that ability and I am asking you to help me to use your ability in a very simple way. Provided that you just follow my simple instructions, there is nothing to stop you achieving a state of hypnosis. The only thing that can stop you is if you choose to resist, but you did not come here today for that, did you? It is true that everybody with an IQ of over 80 can be hypnotised and I can see that you are far cleverer than that so that is fine, is it not?"

If you as a therapist would like to have a better understanding of the use of the many strategies that can be employed to induce hypnosis, I would recommend that you buy a copy of *The New Encyclopaedia of Stage Hypnotism*. This is the work of the 'Dean of American Hypnotism', Ormond McGill, and contains the representation of a lifetime in the field of hypnosis.

After the Session

Having terminated the trance, the client should be allowed a few moments to completely re-orientate himself then he should leave promtly as we do not wish to give him the opportunity to rationalise the session content.

I explain to him that, because of his smoking, he has accumulated many toxins and chemicals in the tissues of his body that need to be flushed out. I recommend that he drink plenty of fluid, at least an extra litre and a half a day, to get his kidneys working in order to eat plenty of fruit or take vitamin tablets. Nicotine destroys vitamin C, and the immune system recovers so much more quickly if the client takes extra at this stage.

"I want you to take an audiotape with you". "This tape is designed to compound the good work that we have done here today". "Listen to it at least once a day for a minimum of two weeks and, after that, if you need it". "The tape will help to strengthen and renew your resolve and ensure that you do not become complacent".

I also furnish the client with a leaflet on the subject. It relates the dangers of smoking in some detail and will remind the client of just why he is making this commitment to himself. The content of this leaflet, entitled 'Freedom From Tobacco', follows on the next page. It is reasonable to assume that the literature that is taken away from the office by our now non-smoker client will find its way into the hands of others who may well become new clients.

Having at this point, been paid, it is time to encourage him to leave with the exhortation to call in after one week to, "let me know how well you are doing".

Freedom from Tobacco

The day that you gave up smoking will rate as one of the most significant of your life, if only for the fact that your life will be longer and of enhanced quality. It is a fact that smokers are now readily accepting the real threat of early death and a very significant reduction in their potential to enjoy good health and all the pleasures that can bring.

It is with our bodies that we enjoy the good things of life, and it has to be folly in the extreme to treat that body with less than the respect and consideration required.

During your therapy session you had the opportunity to look realistically at what smoking has meant to you and to accept fully the responsibility that is yours to ensure that you do not deliberately poison yourself.

We began with finding out why you started smoking. Usually, and with only rare exceptions, it began with 'peer pressure'.

Over the years the advertising of cigarettes has been targeted at the young. The suggestions that are levelled at those just at the gate of adulthood are insidious and cruel, levelled by people who have great power to ensure that their message is heard.

Their thought is for profit and profit alone without any consideration for the harm that they inflict on their fellow members of the human race. Cigarettes have killed more people in the twentieth century than in all the wars and conflicts.

Advertising suggests that it is 'cool' to smoke; that it is a mark of becoming more adult, more sophisticated. In our formative years we are in so much of a rush to become adult and we can be so naive.

Remember the first cigarette; how foul it tasted; how dizzy you felt. Perhaps you felt sick? You certainly did not enjoy it, but in the drive to be seen as one of the crowd ... more sophisticated and adult, so you persisted and you became hooked.

So what happened? Why did your body become at first tolerant of your efforts to poison it and then dependent on your continuing to the point of addiction?

The chemical make-up of the body is balanced and critical. It is the job of the subconscious mind to ensure that all is well and that the necessary functions of the body are regulated.

When the first smoke entered into your lungs it carried with it a myriad of poisonous and noxious compounds. Some you are familiar with, such as tar and nicotine.

What of substances such as cyanide, arsenic, carbon monoxide, prussic acid, benzo-pyrene and ammonia, and then the chemical fertilisers and insecticides that were sprayed onto the crop?

Cyanide – that grabbed your attention. Well it would, but what about nicotine? Are you aware that nicotine is one of the most poisonous substances known to man? The nicotine extracted from one cigarette, if injected directly into a vein, will kill you in seconds. It is enough to kill a horse.

Your body reacted to these poisons by trying to expel them as it made you feel nauseous. The dizziness was caused by the fact that you had deprived your brain of oxygen, and the coughing as your lungs' defence system became activated, trying to cough up and expel the foreign matter that was attempting to contaminate them.

It is the job of the subconscious mind to protect the integrity of the body and in doing this it will give you a reminder when you are feeling hungry or thirsty; it will let you know when you need to visit the toilet. It ensures that when you are asleep your heart and other organs continue to function. You have no need to be conscious of your heart beating, or that your kidneys and your liver are quietly doing their essential work. All is regulated and controlled for your benefit by your subconscious.

In an attempt to regulate and preserve the delicate chemical balance, the subconscious provided you with plenty of signals as it told you that you were poisoning yourself. Yet you persisted, and it came to the point where the subconscious became fooled into thinking that the new and noxious chemicals being introduced through the cigarette smoke were necessary for survival and now, in keeping with its function, messages began to be sent for replenishment whenever the level of nicotine dropped. Here we have the beginning of nicotine addiction.

These messages are the craving that is experienced which have encouraged you to light up another cigarette to preserve the new chemical balance now considered to be correct by your subconscious. In trying to do its best for you it was encouraging you to continue a process that causes great harm to every organ of your body.

When you introduce cigarette smoke into your body, it reacts in the same manner as it would if you were confronted with something terrifying. The body goes into 'Fight or flight mode' as it prepares itself to deal with imminent danger.

The heart beats faster, respiration increases as the need for oxygen to the muscles and the brain increases. Adrenaline is produced along with lactic acid to increase the readiness of the muscles to respond with rapid reaction as you either fight or run from the danger. **So many people have told me that a cigarette helps them to relax. It hardly seems likely!**

As these things happen the body also shuts down those systems that will not be needed during this period of increased readiness for survival action. The digestive system is not required so it is shut down, and the immune system is also not required during this time so it too is shut down.

In normal situations of danger the period during which the body remains in the fight or flight mode is brief. When the danger is past then the body reverts to its normal relaxation mode, and there is no problem.

But when we continue to smoke there is no opportunity for the body to revert from the flight or fight mode to the normal relaxation mode. The stress is constant, and so the body remains on alert. Now smokers are in real danger. Those enzymes produced to enhance performance are not used in running or fighting and so remain as toxins within the body.

It is small wonder that those who smoke are more susceptible to disease than non- smokers. With their immune system constantly suppressed they do not have the ability to ward off infection, and so when the cold and flu viruses are about they are the first to fall victim and they are also the last to shake of the effects of the virus. Of course a cold is the least that need concern us.

The horror word amongst smokers, the word that none dare speak, is, of course, cancer. "It won't happen to me. Cancer only happens to other people". This is our subconscious speaking to reassure us because it really does think now that smoking is something we need to do to ensure that our bodily integrity is maintained with sufficient in the way of poison.

Cancer is within us all if the production of new cells is somehow allowed to run out of control, and then the problems begin. What ensures that we avoid this is the functioning of an ever alert and healthy immune system. When our defences are down we are more vulnerable to attack.

Vitamin C is important for the maintenance of the immune system. Nicotine destroys Vitamin C.

Every organ of the body, including the brain and the skin, can fall to cancer, and smoking has to be seen as a major culprit in the body's inability to protect itself against this and many other killer diseases.

The heart of a smoker will beat an extra 10,000 beats a day as it strives to combat the effects of nicotine which is recognised as a vaso constrictor. The arteries narrow under its influence, and so the heart has to work so much harder to pump the blood around those arteries which are also subject to the effects of furring up as the filth and muck is pumped around them, causing arteriosclerosis.

Increased blood pressure is, of course, the result, and with it comes the heightened risk of heart disease and heart attack.

Blood carries vital oxygen to every organ, every molecule and every cell of the body. Without oxygen, tissue will simply dies. Mortification of the flesh sets in – to give it a name that is familiar – gangrene.

Because of the effects of smoking the tissues furthest from the heart become deprived of vital oxygen and so, in order to save your life, the surgeon will cut off your leg – perhaps both. Where is the quality of life now?

It is the function of the lungs to oxygenate the blood. The airways that lead into the lungs are covered with tiny hair-line projections called cilia. It is their function to detect the ingress of any foreign matter such as particles of dust which they then propel back upwards to the mouth, thus expelling any harmful material.

The tar in cigarettes coats these tiny hairs with a thick sticky residue which causes them to become brittle, to break off or to lie flat against the walls of the airways. They are thus no longer able to carry out this so important defence function.

The chemicals within the smoke affect to great detriment the mucus lining of the lungs that is so important in the vital interchange of gases, carbon dioxide and oxygen.

Tar and other materials pass unhindered down into the small air spaces called alveoli which make up the greater mass of the lungs and accumulate there. They remain there, and so the capacity of the lungs is reduced and consequently the ability to efficiently oxygenate the blood.

You will now understand why smokers get out of breath when tackling stairs or running for a bus. You may have seen the horror pictures of a smoker's lungs on TV, but then your subconscious helped you to dissociate yourself from that too. Remember, it really has been deceived into believing that it must ensure that you get your nicotine fix for your health.

The effect of chemically altering the mucus lining of the lungs has an awful and debilitating effect for some as the lungs produce too much fluid and then begin to fill up. The people unlucky enough to be so afflicted begin to drown slowly in their own body fluids.

Emphysema is a word that becomes for these poor souls a nightmare as they fight for every painful breath, an oxygen cylinder constantly at their side, with only one possible outcome.

It has been established that the effect of smoking can affect the genetic pattern within the sperm of the male and the eggs of the female, the DNA, the building blocks of life. It is also true that reproductive potency is detrimentally affected. Humans are sexual animals, and one of the main pleasures of life is that of normal sexual relations. The sexual prowess of a smoker will decrease at a much faster rate than that of a non-smoker. Thus in order to enjoy sex, it follows that we must be the best that we can be, fit and healthy, free of contaminants and poisons so that we can give of our best. That means being a non-smoker!

Every cigarette that you smoke will rob you of up to six minutes of life expectancy. A fifty-year-old smoker is as old physically as a seventy-year-old non-smoker. Such are the effects of poisoning your body day in, day out.

You have already reached the conclusion that this is not your way forward and as you listen to the tape that is provided with your therapy, the message to your subconscious will be continually strengthened and compounded for your benefit.

Do not allow yourself to become complacent. The advice given is that you listen to the tape regularly for at least two weeks and at least once every day. I know it may be boring but so is death and disease, and remember too that this is a period of re-education for your subconscious as it re-learns to protect you from what it previously thought was right for you. Until this re-education is complete your subconscious will continue to try misguidedly to do its old job and will try every trick in the book to get you to submit.

Listen to side 'B' of the tape as you drive your car or while you go about your normal daily life. The subliminal messages are powerful and will continue to drive home positive affirmations to ensure that the work of re-education is thoroughly done.

You have been advised that, in order to flush out the accumulated rubbish from within your body, you need to drink plenty. A litre of water a day is the minimum you should be drinking and, if you find yourself constantly leaping up to go to the toilet, then that is great – the job is being done in the most natural and effective way.

Soon you begin to experience the things that you have missed as a smoker. Your clothes and your hair smell fresh. You taste the food that you eat so much more, and the perfume of the summer flowers will delight you with its intensity.

Your energy levels will rise, and you will become and feel so much more in control of your life and so much more attractive as a person. You will notice that the condition of your skin and your hair improves. Your eyesight becomes clearer as the oxygen levels within your blood become normal and then, as your brain receives its full quota of oxygen, you will think so much more clearly. A smoker on twenty cigarettes a day loses up to 23% of clear thinking ability simply because the brain has been deprived of oxygen.

Who said that a cigarette aids concentration?

When you are thinking so clearly, you will think with the utmost clarity, "Why on earth did I start in the first place?" Did I mention all the money that has gone up in smoke?

My parting words have become a habit as people leave my office after their session, and I make no excuse for using this phrase, "Go and sin no more". You are now fully aware of your responsibility for your own life, health and happiness and accept that it is your responsibility to ensure that those who love you and rely on you are not deprived of that special person through crass stupidity.

Congratulations on your excellent achievement as you say with pride in your accomplishment, "**I am a non-smoker**".

The benefits of quitting or reducing your cigarette smoking can be tremendous, especially if you have smoked less than 10 pack years. (i.e. the equivalent of smoking a pack a day for 10 years.) Even if you have smoked more than that the benefits will still outweigh the challenges.

Aaaaaahhhhh smoking! Gasp-wheeze-cough-choke! Oh, that was so hard to say! (damaged voice ... no wind ... depletion of energy) Ooooh, how I hate it! This thief has managed to damage almost every fibre of my life: my character, my desire to show love to others and my ability to serve God. It has robbed me of so many of the things I cherish! Like being with people, laughing, singing, talking, hugging, kissing, cuddling, sitting near to comfort or talk intimately with someone I care about. It has forced me to be less affectionate, less expressive, less tender. Smelly people can't do these 'feely' types of things freely. (you can't hug someone if they get nauseated by your smell!) **No one told me it would be like this when I started to smoke!**

Smoking denies me so many freedoms! Not only the freedom to love others at will or burst into song, but also, the freedom to laugh at a good joke or cry during a sad movie. I can no longer do these things as smoking has damaged my vocal cords. (Oh, how I hate the sound of my own deep, raspy, wheezy, harsh voice – a smoker's voice. Everyone can recognise a smoker by it.) When I want to express tenderness or gentleness with my voice, I can't. I always sound angry or harsh. I want to be able to use my voice to express the way I feel, but my voice won't let me because of smoking, and **no one told me it would be like this when I started to smoke!**

It has stolen my freedom to go places that I long to go to or to join in with others, at will, for fun activities like vacations, conferences, trips to the city to shop or whatever my friends are up to. I am unable to go away on trips with friends, drive any distance in a car with them to concerts, games, events etc. I am unable to stay in their homes or share a motel room with them. Smoking has not only made me an unaccepted, disrespected person (for smoking is offensive for non-smokers), it has forced me to become a recluse. Something I hate! Sometimes I feel a need to hide from others out of shame and embarrassment or simply to avoid hearing another lecture on why smoking is no good for me (as though I don't know that already!). I have found that I don't handle very well seeing their repulsion or comments at the sight of me smoking. I know they have less respect for me when they see me smoke and they are truly disappointed in me. Children seem to be really affected by it. It breaks their hearts to see me smoke, but **no one told me it would be like this when I started to smoke!**

I feel it is rude to smoke in front of someone while in their home, in their car or even while just sitting at a sporting event with them. Therefore I have learned to avoid these types of situations. I don't want to offend or insult them or hurt them with my second-hand smoke. I don't want to be rude and, since I can't go more than a few hours without a smoke, I just **don't** go! It makes me feel so left out all the time. I miss out on so much fun ... **why didn't anyone tell me about all the things I would be left out of when I started to smoke!**

Health issues? You're probably aware of cancer, heart disease, emphysema, etc, but have you ever considered the real heart issues at stake here? The isolation, the loneliness and the sadness a smoker feels because he smokes? The rejection, the hurt and the embarrassment he feels by being a smoker? The good times lost or the missed chances to go places and be with people he loves?

But the real clincher is: have you ever wanted to sing a lullaby to your child, but couldn't? Or whisper sweet nothings in your husband's ear, but couldn't? Or touch someone's face gently and say I care about you, but couldn't? Lost moments, lost memories, lost chances to say **I love you**, all because of smoking! **No one told me it would be like this when I started to smoke!**

As far as I can tell, there is **only** one good thing about the fact that I am a smoker, and that is that I have the right and the confidence to stand up and be a **wild waving red flag** of warning to others who consider starting. **If** I could scream, without a gasp-wheeze-cough-choke, you'd hear me hollering at the top of my lungs, "**Don't smoke!! Don't even play with the stuff! You will regret it for as long as you live, I guarantee it!**"

I hope someday, somewhere, someone will be able to say, "**I listened and believed what someone told me about smoking, things I didn't know before and that is why I never started!**" And that would be good.

When you stop smoking:

- **Within 20 Minutes:** Your blood pressure and pulse rate drop to normal, and the body temperature of your hands and feet increases to normal.
- **Within 8 Hours:** The carbon monoxide level in your blood drops to normal and the oxygen level in you blood increases to normal.
- **Within 24 Hours:** Your chances of having a heart attack already decreases.
- **Within 48 Hours:** Your nerve endings start to grow and your sense of smell and taste improve.
- **Within 72 Hours:** Your bronchial tubes begin to relax and you can breathe more easily. Your lung capacity also increases which means that you can do more physical activities more easily.
- **Within 2 Weeks to 3 Months:** Your circulation improves, walking becomes easier and your lung function increases by up to 30 per cent.
- **Within 1 Month to 9 Months:** Coughing, sinus congestion, fatigue and shortness of breath continue to decrease and your overall level of energy increases. The cilia re-grow in your lungs thus increasing your ability to handle mucus and to clean out your lungs and to reduce infection.
- **At 5 Years:** The lung cancer death rate drops.
- **At 10 Years:** The lung cancer death rate for the average smoker drops to 12 deaths per I0,0000, almost the rate of non-smokers. Other cancers, such as those of the mouth, larynx, oesophagus, bladder, kidneys and pancreas also decrease. (Remember, there are 30 chemicals in tobacco smoke that cause cancer.) Pre-cancerous cells are replaced.

Every November we as a nation pause for a moment to remember those who lost their lives fighting in the great wars that have marred the twentieth century. Human beings fighting each other in the name of what? The answer has to be the vested interest of a few who not content with their power and wealth, who seek more and spare no thought for those who die in the struggle.

Man fighting man is much like the smoker fighting him or herself for the right to quit. There will be losses on both side of the conflict. Even the victor suffers loss. In giving up smoking you can be on the winning or the losing side. The losing side suffers greatly through loss of life and in suffering. The winning side also suffers, through withdrawal, but emerges victorious over the greater evil that is smoking.

Plan for yourself a memorial day to celebrate your own victory over cigarettes and the death of your insidious and destructive habit. Celebrate your triumph over the tobacco companies, before others have to honour your memory at your graveside.

The Battle Won?

The client has gone from the office, having received all the warnings and feeling that nothing can deter him – that his battle is won.

The enemy is not dead and begins now a guerrilla war within to regain the strength that will diminish in time as the non-smoker grows more powerful. He can lie in wait for years, just waiting for the opportunity to pounce unexpectedly at a party perhaps, or when life presents a difficulty.

"Go on. Just one won't hurt ... you can stop whenever you want to."

"You will feel more part of the group if you just have a cigarette with them."

"A gorgeous member of the opposite sex, obviously interested in you, offers you a cigarette." The subconscious smoker will turn up the hormones that control the sexual urges and it will seem as nothing to just have a cigarette to achieve that sexual conquest.

"You are so sad. Remember how a cigarette used to make you feel better?"

"A cigarette will keep those midges away."

A smoker is in the same boat as a recovering alcoholic. He can never smoke again because that one cigarette is all that is needed to revive that sleeping enemy within, 'the subconscious smoker', just waiting to grab the opportunity. Just one that will not hurt is the one that will begin the sorry story all over again. Remember that it all began with just one cigarette.

The Audiotape

I use an audiotape that I have recorded myself. The fact that the client is hearing my voice when listening to it enhances the message. I will have suggested to him before he left my office that listening to the tape, to the sound of my voice, will serve to strengthen all the work that was done in the therapy session.

This is side 'A' of the tape and contains a hypnotic induction, and should only be listened to when relaxing comfortably. Side 'B' contains music within which subliminal positive affirmations are imbedded. This side can be listened to at any time, even when driving or when operating machinery and constantly feeds the positive messages direct to the subconscious.

The tape is useful in that it contains suggestions that strengthen the work done in the office. The client understands this and realises that the therapeutic benefits will be on-going provided he listens to the audiotape.

The content of side 'A' of the tape is "the Diamond Smoking Script" found in *Scripts and Strategies in Hypnotherapy* by this author and available from the publishers of this book. I would add that I was in fact pleasantly surprised at the many accolades that came my way after the publication of this volume and suggest that it would prove a useful part of any therapist's library. Commercial concluded!

While on the subject of post-therapy aids, I would mention that there are on the market many video tapes that are designed to help smokers to quit. Many, I feel, are of dubious worth but there is one video programme available in the UK that is part of a series or library of therapeutic video programmes known as Psychovisual Therapy. The 'Stop Smoking' video is excellent and has the distinction of having received accolades from the British Medical Council and from The Life Assurance Trust as being the most effective video programme of its kind. I myself have used these videos and am greatly impressed by them. Each of the programmes consists of no less than twelve therapeutic strategies that also incorporate powerful visual images and relaxing music while the voice-over delivers both overt and covert positive messages. Flowing computer generated colours and shapes relax the viewer into a light trance during which the subconscious can absorb the subliminal messages more readily.

(*Most PsyV programmes also include overt information delivered through a combination of voice-over and illustrations. Specially created music relaxes the viewer, as do the computer-generated images, so that the subliminal messages are absorbed that much more easily. Carr-Jones 1992*)

Those who have internet facilities may wish to log onto the webpage: http://poole.internet.co.uk/videos.html. If you do not have this facility and wish to know more about Psychovisual Therapy, I am sure that Michael Carr-Jones will be delighted if you give him a call. He is an eminently respected hypnotherapist and practises in Poole, Dorset. Tel: +44 (0)1202 739369.
E-mail: michaelcarrjones@aol.com

Now I have come to the end of this book, I sincerely hope that my efforts will be of some value to you. This work is the amalgamation of many others over the years. I have tried to give accreditation wherever possible, but like so many before me, I can only apologise to all those who have contributed to the great mass of knowledge encompassed within the profession who I cannot bring to mind. I trust that my thanks to all who have influenced me will be accepted.

Bibliography

Allen, Roger. P (1997) *Scripts and Strategies in Hypnotherapy.* Carmarthen, Wales, UK: Crown House Publishing.

Andreas, Connirae & Steve. (1987) *Change Your Mind—and Keep the Change.* Moab, Utah, USA: Real People Press.

Bandler, Richard. (1985) *Using Your Brain—For A Change.* Moab, Utah, USA: Real People Press.

Havens, Ronald & Walters, Catherine. (1989) *Hypnotherapy Scripts: A Neo-Ericksonian Approach to Persuasive Healing.* New York, USA: Brunner/Mazel.

Kennedy, Eugene & Charles, Sara C. (1991) *On Becoming a Counsellor: A Basic Guide for Non-Professional Counsellors.* Dublin, Ireland: Gill and Macmillan.

Knight, Bryan M. & Carr-Jones, Michael. (1992) *Love Sex & Hypnosis.* The Chestnut Press.

Narramore, Clyde Maurice. (1966) *Encyclopaedia of Psychological Problems, Second Edition.* Edinburgh, UK: Marshall, Morgan & Scott.

Tebbetts, Charles. (1987) *Self Hypnosis and Other Mind Expanding Techniques.* Glendale, California: Westwood Publishing Company, Inc.

Walker, Stephen.(1984) *Learning Theory and Behaviour Modification.* London, UK: Methuen.

Williams, Edward Lincoln. (1967) *Alcoholism Explained.* London, UK: Evans Brothers Ltd.

Yapko, Michael D. (1990) *Trancework: An Introduction to the Practice of Clinical Hypnosis, Second Edition.* New York, USA: Brunner/Mazel.

Videotape Acknowledgements

Stop Smoking. Psychological Research and Development Organisation Ltd.